Ketogenic Diet Recipes

155+ low-carb recipes for weight loss beginners

Maria Travis

continued validity or interim quality. Trademarks that mentioned are done without written consent and can in no way be considered an endorsement from the trademark holder.

Description

Weight loss is possible and you can do it rapidly if you follow the ketogenic diet. It is one of the simplest, most effective and quickest diets for you to choose to follow and it will give you a chance to see dramatic results in a short period of time.

Not only does this book include what you need to know about the diet, but it also includes the information that you need to know about how to start it, the meal plans and the recipes that you will be able to use.

Included in the book is information regarding:

- The way the ketogenic diet works
- How you can use it for different health issues
- A plethora of recipes that are keto-friendly

Are you ready to get healthy and treat your body to the food it deserves?

Table of Contents

Introduction

Congratulations on downloading your personal copy of *Ketogenic Diet Recipes: 155+ low-carb recipes for weight loss beginners*. Thank you for doing so.

The following chapters will discuss some of the many recipes that you can use with the ketogenic diet beginning you being able to learn a lot of information about the diet.

You will discover how important it is to make sure that you are getting what you can and getting nearly perfect nutrition from the recipes.

The final chapter will also explore fun drink recipes that you can use for your ketogenic diet.

There are plenty of books on this subject on the market, thanks again for choosing this one! Every effort was made to ensure it is full of as much useful information as possible. Enjoy!

Part 1:

Learning About

the

Ketogenic Diet

Chapter 1:

The Basics of Ketogenic Diet

While the ketogenic diet seems relatively simple (eat good fats, avoid Net carbohydrates, etc.), it comes from both science and biology because of the way that people are able to process different types of nutrition. There are many ways to do the diet, but most the ways rely on you being able to cut out Net carbohydrates as soon as possible; the sooner that you cut out carbohydrates, the sooner you will be able to enter ketosis and start losing weight.

But what, exactly, is ketosis?

Ketosis

The state in which you burn fat from your body, instead of food that you are putting into your body right then, is called "ketosis." This is the state that your body enters just before starvation but it is not nearly as detrimental and it is not as harmful to the body.

Because of the way that ketosis works, you will need to make sure that you are "resetting" your system, meaning you will need to enter the point where you switch from burning the fuel that you eat as food and change the fuel that you are using as your body fat.

If you can enter Ketosis, you will start to lose weight. This is because your body will survive on the fat that is on your body (which, by the way, is the point of *having* fat). You will need to do the diet for a few days before you enter ketosis but as soon as you get to that point, you will continue to lose weight for the entire length of time that you are cutting out the Net carbohydrates in your diet. It is necessary to be able to stay in ketosis if you want to keep losing weight.

High Fat

Since you will not be eating Net carbohydrates, you need to do something that will prevent you from entering starvation mode. As you have already learned in the previous paragraphs, starvation mode is bad for your body while ketosis is good.

To be able to keep your body in ketosis and out of starvation, you need to make sure that you are eating something that will help you to stay as nourished as possible. Eating a diet that is high in fat is what will allow you the chance to be able to make sure that you are going to stay as nourished as possible. It is a good idea to keep yourself full so that you will not want to cheat and eat food that is not allowed.

While fat has generally been looked at as "bad" nutrition, it is no longer thought of that way. While there are good and bad fats that are present in different foods, you need to make sure that you are eating fat to keep yourself as full as possible. It will keep you satisfied whereas the problems that normally would come from fat actually come from eating both fat and carbohydrates together.

Average Protein

While other diets that are low in Net carbohydrates focus on protein, the ketogenic diet focuses the majority of your nutrition on fatty foods. Since fats and proteins normally go hand in hand, there is no real reason for you to try to limit protein because that is something that will help keep you away from carbohydrates just as much as what the fats will do.

Even though you will need to make sure that you are eating a lot of food that is high in fat, you will also need to eat an average amount of protein. Eating protein will give you a great chance at staying full and being able to "hold yourself" over until it is time for the next meal.

When you are looking for protein sources that you are going to eat while you are doing the ketogenic diet, you need to make sure that you are trying to find food that is both full of protein and fat. Fats that are higher in protein will be the best options for you when you are doing more with your diet.

There is no need for low-fat protein in the ketogenic diet.

Low / No Net Carbohydrates

When you first start out with the ketogenic diet, your carb intake will be strictly limited. This can be difficult for some people, but it is necessary to make sure that you are going to be able to truly get the best experience. Your body will need to "detox" from Net carbohydrates, especially if you have been used to Net carbohydrates in the past.

As you progress throughout the diet, you will need to make some changes to your diet so that you can connect with the changes that you have. For example, you will need to try new things with the Net carbohydrates that you are eating. When you get close to the end of the diet, or are where you want to be with your goals, you will need to make sure that you are adding Net carbohydrates back slowly. The maintenance phase of the keto diet will allow you to eat some Net carbohydrates, but you must keep in mind that carbohydrates are bad for your body; they do not bring a high level of nutrition and they can sometimes be dangerous for your body if your diet is made up of mostly Net carbohydrates.

Sustainability

Unlike some diets that are available for weight loss, the ketogenic diet is something that you will be able to do for a long time. The ketogenic diet was designed to be sustainable, and something that you could rely on regardless of your weight loss goals. If you are going to do the ketogenic diet, you will need to make sure that you are prepared for a lifetime of commitment because the diet is something that you will want to stick with for the rest of your life.

The way that keto is designed is so that you can go through different phases and stages of the diet. While you are very limited in the Net carbohydrates that you can eat at the beginning, as you go through the diet, you will be allowed to eat more Net carbohydrates; this is to help teach you the way that you can eat Net carbohydrates healthily and how you can make the right choices for your Net carbohydrates.

There is no other diet that is designed to teach you *how* to add back in the "bad" foods to your diet so that you will be able to enjoy them without being so restricted for the rest of your life. Keep that in mind while you are doing keto and you will be able to truly eat the right way in the future.

Ease of Diet

Dieting is hard. There is no way around that and you will have to make some major life changes no matter what diet you are planning on doing. However, you will be able to make the most out of the diet that you are doing when you use the ketogenic diet.

While there is no diet that is going to be easy because you need to change your lifestyle, the ketogenic diet is something that you will find easy compared to other diets. As far as diets are concerned, the ketogenic diet is one of the easiest things that you can do and it will help you to lose the weight that you need to be able to change the way that you live.

As you are going through the different phases of the diet, you will need to make sure that you are doing what you can. The phases not only teach you how to add Net Carbohydrates back into your diet but it will also help you to figure out what your life is going to look forward to later on in the diet. As you are doing more with your diet, you will make the most out of the choices that you have. You will learn which Net Carbohydrates work best with your body and what you can eat without getting out of hand.

Keep all the aspects in mind while you are doing different things on the diet. Whether you are planning the meals that you are going to make, shopping for the ingredients or making the recipes, you should be aware that you are going to be able to truly benefit from a high fat, low-carb diet.

Chapter 2:

Steps of the Ketogenic Diet

As with any diet, there are steps that you will need to follow with the ketogenic diet to ensure that you are getting the best nutrition and the best chance possible at actually being able to lose weight. As you learn more about the diet and the different aspects of it, you will find that the steps are all easy, and that you can lose weight easily if you just follow each of the steps.

One thing that you should keep in mind is that every person is different. While it may take one person several months to get through one step, it may take another person only a few weeks until they are in the next part of the diet. If you want to make sure that you are getting the best ketogenic experience possible, you will need to make sure that you ease yourself into the diet and go slowly so that you can make sure that you are used to the diet. It will give you a chance to be able to do more with it and to try more with the diet.

Prepping Yourself

This is the most important part of the diet and will determine whether you will do well or you will fail at the ketogenic diet. You need to not only prepare yourself physically for the requirements of the diet by getting the food that you will be able to eat, but you also need to make sure that you are preparing yourself mentally for the diet and what it is going to be able to do to help you.

Some of the things that you can do:

- Go shopping for no / low-carb foods

- Create a meal plan for yourself
- Write down all of the goals that you have for the diet
- Understand that *right now* is the right time to start (there is no perfect timing for diets)
- Learn as much about the body and the diet as possible

As you go through the different steps of the diet preparation, you will notice that there are many things that you can do to help yourself get the best experience possible. This doesn't necessarily mean that you will not be able to start the diet, but it will help you to have a better chance at succeeding with it.

Easing into It

The idea behind easing into the diet is something that works for some people but does not for others. This is because people have different personalities and different eating habits that are associated with those personalities. If you think that easing into the diet will be difficult for you, simply start "cold turkey" and cut out all the Net carbohydrates that you are eating.

If you want to try "easing" into the diet, you can try to cut out certain types of Net carbohydrates so that you will be able to try new things and see that there is more than just the basic Net carbohydrates that you might be used to.

If you want to ease into the diet, start by cutting out bread. Then, cut out some other types of processed Net carbohydrates like crackers, pretzels, and other snacks. After you have done that, you can cut out other types of Net carbohydrates like starchy vegetables and fruits that can sabotage your sugar goals while you are doing the ketogenic diet.

Getting Started

If you are done easing into the diet, or, if you have chosen to skip right to this step, you will need to make sure that you are cutting out *all* Net carbohydrates in your diet. Look for things that have hidden Net carbohydrates and things that are going to harm your diet. Throw away the Net carbohydrates that you have in your home whether they are cans of corn or boxes of pasta; they are going to hurt your diet, so get rid of them right now before you even get started with the rest of the diet. You will be able to benefit more from each of these things and help yourself while you are getting started.

Keep in mind that you will feel very hungry in the first few days of the diet. Even if you have eased into it, completely cutting out Net carbohydrates can be somewhat difficult, but you should know that you are going to be able to do it if you just stick with it. It is important that you try to make sure that you are going to get the diet done.

When you get hungry, have things that are easy for you to reach for so that you don't reach for the bag of chips. Things that you can munch on in the first few days:

- Pickles
- Beef jerky
- "Fat Bombs"
- Cream cheese
- Cloud bread
- Cubes of cheese
- Snack meats – chicken and beef bites

Your Exercise Routine

You didn't think that you would get away with losing weight without adding *any* type of exercise in, did you? While it is possible to do the ketogenic diet without exercising, you will

9

not get the best results possible. If you want to truly enjoy the different aspects of the diet and lose a lot of weight, you will need to do some form of exercise.

Similar to when you started dieting, make sure that you do it slowly and do not push yourself too hard to start an exercise routine. You will need to make sure that you are doing what you can to make the routine better. After you have been doing the diet for a month or two, you can start adding exercise in. The best plan to do while you are eating a low-carb diet is a high-intensity interval training program. This means that you will do a different exercise each day of the week. The exercises should be a difficult level, but they should be short. By doing these short bursts of different exercise, you will not allow your muscles to get "used" to any single exercise that you might be doing.

Active Weight Loss

Throughout the bulk of the diet, you will have active weight loss. This is the most important part of the diet, and it will continue to work for you if you are following it the right way. While plateaus are uncommon while doing the ketogenic diet, there is a chance that you could have a plateau. At that point, you should not change anything about your diet (other than checking to see if you have hidden Net carbohydrates in anything you are eating), but you should change your exercise routine.

Doing this will allow you the chance to make sure that you are going to get the best experience possible and that you are going to be able to try new things with your weight loss. It is important that you are going to get the best experience possible and that you are going to be able to try more with the diet that you are doing. If you want to be able to truly enjoy the diet, you will need to maintain active weight loss for as long as you are doing it.

Reaching Your Goals

As you get closer to the goal weight that you want to be, you may notice that your weight loss is slowing down. This is because your body is getting accustomed to the diet and it knows that it has reached a very healthy weight so that it will be able to perform in the best way possible. If you want to keep losing weight, you will still need to stick with the diet that you have done throughout this time so that you can make sure that you are going to get the most amount of weight loss.

The goal that you have set yourself is just a goal – if you get there and you find that you have not lost what you wanted to lose, or that your health snapshot does not look like you want it to, consider trying different things to help you get the best experience possible. You can always add more goals to the ones that you already have and that will give you a chance to be able to truly reach where you want to be.

Keep in mind that your goal weight is not the end of the line; you will still have to maintain your weight loss.

Maintaining

Some people who have dieted have actually said that maintenance is the hardest part of the diet because of the problems that come from thinking that you are going to be able to just go back to your old eating habits. Since you are trying new things with your weight loss and you are going to be able to do more with it, you will need to make sure that you are doing what you can to continue to lose weight. For some people, that means that they are going to have to try new things during maintenance.

While you are maintaining your weight, make sure that you do not eat too many Net carbohydrates and that you do not try too hard to lose weight. Your body and hormones should level out when you are an appropriate weight, so that will help you have the best experience possible while also give you the chance to be able to maintain the weight that you are at. It is detrimental not to do so.

Adding Net Carbohydrates Back In

After you have been maintaining your weight loss for a period of time, you may want to consider adding Net carbohydrates back into your diet. This is the only thing that you can do to add Net carbohydrates back in – add *good* Net carbohydrates like fruit and some starchy vegetables. Be careful how much you are adding, and always keep track of your weight in the beginning so that you will know how much and what you can add back in without gaining weight. It is important to make sure that you are going to get the best type of nutrition from your Net carbohydrates, so the majority of them should come from fruit.

Try to avoid processed Net carbohydrates no matter what. While the occasional slice of wheat bread will not cause you to gain 100 pounds back onto your waistline, it is best to avoid them when you can. You can get all the Net carbohydrates that you need from fruit, vegetables, and other sources that have them in them. While some processed meats, like sausage, have Net carbohydrates in them and are heavily processed, it is not the worst thing that you can eat. Fat and Net carbohydrates work well together while you are maintaining your weight loss.

Weight Gain?

If at any time during the diet, you find that you are gaining weight and you are still dieting, you need to check a few things.

The most obvious thing would be that there are secret Net carbohydrates in something that you eat. Salami, summer sausage, and even bologna sometimes have Net carbohydrates in them. Check that information out and be sure that you eliminate them from your diet if you find that they have hidden Net carbohydrates.

Other things that could be causing problems are that you are not getting *enough* fat. If you are not getting an appropriate amount of nutrition to help fuel your body, it may be in starvation mode. This can cause you to not be able to lose weight or even gain weight while you are dieting. This can be a huge problem if you want to make sure that you are losing weight; keep in mind that you need to adjust your diet so that you are getting the right amount of fat and protein to provide fuel to yourself.

It is a good idea to keep track of what you are eating. You may find that you are not eating enough to keep your body fueled up.

Chapter 3:

Meal Plans for the Ketogenic Diet

Meal planning is one of the easiest ways that you can be successful when you are doing any type of diet. The ketogenic diet is no different, and using the meal plans that are provided will help you have a more enjoyable diet experience. It will also give you a chance to be able to do more with the diet options that you have. Despite the fact that you can try more things without a meal plan, you will need to make sure that you are doing what you can with the meal plan. Always use your best judgment to be able to use the meal plans.

By taking a closer look at meal plans and what they mean for dieters, you will be able to see the benefits that come along with them. Just make sure that you follow the plans so that you don't have to worry about 1) getting bored with the diet or 2) not knowing what you are going to eat and then eating an entire loaf of bread (don't do that, even if you aren't following the keto diet).

The Benefits

The benefits of using a meal plan come with the fact that you will be able to have a much easier time with the diet that you are doing so that you will be able to try new things with the diets that you have. It will allow you to try new things and get the most out of your meals by showing you what you are going to eat each time that you sit down for a meal.

Along with the benefits that come with seeing what you are going to eat ahead of time, you will be able to see benefits in the fact that it is easier not to have to make a decision right before you eat a meal. The chances that you are going to choose a good and nutritious meal that you have planned ahead of time are much better when you have the meal plan that tells you what you are going to do; it is a great way to ensure that you will be successful with the ketogenic diet.

Proven Success

There are many studies that have been performed that show that you will be more successful with *any* diet that you do when you are able to plan ahead for that diet. Planning is important in every aspect of life, but is especially so when you are eating in a way that will allow you to try and make the most out of the food that you eat. Your nutrition will be much easier for you to handle when you know what you are going to eat ahead of time and don't have to make split-second decisions on what the dinner plan is.

For a meal plan to actually be able to work, you will need to make sure that you are sticking to it. There is no point in making a menu for the week and planning for that menu if you are not going to be able to do it when the time comes. One thing that many people choose to do is to not only create a meal plan but to also prepare the majority of the meals that they are going to eat throughout the week ahead of time so that it is one less thing that they have to worry about.

An Easier Life

Life is busy for most people, and some just don't have the time to sit down and think about what they are going to make for dinner each day. It is even harder when you factor in work, kids, and all the other aspects of life that can cause you to miss out on the things that you should be doing for your health. When you have a meal plan in place, you will know what you are eating each day and what you need to do to prepare the meal ahead of time.

One of the things that many people do is prepare their meals a week ahead of time. This will allow you to give yourself the chance to do more with the food that you have and with the options that are included in your various meal plans. Keep in mind that all of the recipes that are in this book can be used for meal prep. You can make them up to one week ahead of time and then simply serve them when it is time to eat the meal that they correspond with on your meal plan; some of the recipes will even allow you to freeze them ahead of time.

How Meal Plans Work

A meal plan works by providing you with an opportunity to prepare meals before you do them and without having to worry about the problems that come along with trying new things out and not getting a chance to do a recipe right before you eat it. While you are creating your meal plans, keep in mind that you will need to make them before you can eat them each day. Allot for the amount of time that it is going to take you while you are creating the meals and for the food that you are going to be able to eat.

Each of the recipes is convenient and not only tells you the basic ingredients and instructions, but also the amount of time that it will take you to prepare the recipe so that you can eat it. It is easy to fit into any meal plan when you know the amount of time that it takes to cook and the specific nutrition information that is included with each of the recipes that are listed in this book.

Having a plan for what you are going to eat is one of the easiest ways that you can be successful with *any* diet that you are doing. It is a good idea to have a plan so that you will be able to do more with the time that you have and so that you can make sure that you are going to get the best experience possible. It is essential if you want to be able to do more with the diet and if you want to give yourself the best possible chance of convenience.

The following meal plans are great for different things that you are doing with the diet. They are divided into the beginning, the middle, and the end of the diet so that you will be able to use any of the recipes that are included in this book.

Since there are so many recipes included with the book, you can mix and match the recipes with each of the meal plans. This makes it easier for you to be able to try new things and to make sure that you are not getting bored with the diet. It will also allow you the chance to be able to try new things and to get a better experience out of the diet that you are doing. By using these meal plans, you will give yourself the boost that you need to truly get the best experience possible and lose the most amount of weight possible.

At the Beginning

Every meal plan that you are going to make will look like this with some snacks thrown in there. It is always a good idea to try and keep snacks close by so that you know what you are reaching for and you don't absentmindedly reach for chips instead of trying to eat the fat bombs that you have stored in your fridge.

The recipes are all interchangeable with each phase of the diet. If you are near the end, feel free to throw in some fruits to replace some of the snacks; this will help your body get accustomed to the good kind of Net carbohydrates again so that you will have an easier time as you make your way toward maintenance.

Breakfast: no Net carbohydrates, choose from breakfast recipes

Lunch: choose from lunch recipes

Dinner: choose from dinner recipes

You will need to eat a lot of snacks during the first week that you are doing the diet. Be prepared to eat every two hours or so as you will be hungry.

It is also important to note that you may get some flu-like symptoms from the diet when you start it out by just cutting Net carbohydrates out. This is a withdrawal phase (similar to what other addicts go through), and you will be able to get through it. Once you go through this process, it will be much easier for you to try and do the diet as your body will have gotten rid of the Net carbohydrates that were still present in it. You may still struggle with cravings during the first few weeks of the diet, but they will not be as bad as what you felt at the beginning of the diet.

During the first few weeks, it is important that you eat less than 20 grams of Net carbohydrates per day because you will be entering into ketosis. This is the way that you will lose weight and if you do not do it the right way, you won't have the best kick-start to your diet possible. You need to make sure that you are going to be able to get the best experience possible by not eating any Net carbohydrates if you can avoid it. The Net carbohydrates that you do eat should come from things like cottage cheese and meats. There are not a lot in those, but save your 20 grams per day because the other ones start to build up if you do not pay attention to what you are doing and what you are eating.

While Dieting

All of the recipes are great to use at any phase in the diet and the meal plan will be able to sustain you.

To help you feel like you are not getting bored with the diet, you can do different things to change up the meal plan. This will also help you to only have to buy ingredients for several different meals.

You will be able to eat the same meals every other day of the week, but you can change it up if you want to.

For example, your meal plan can look like this:

Breakfast 1: Monday, Wednesday, Friday, and Sunday
Breakfast 2: Tuesday, Thursday, and Saturday

Lunch 1: Monday, Wednesday, Friday, and Sunday
Lunch 2: Tuesday, Thursday, and Saturday

Dinner 1: Monday, Wednesday, Friday, and Sunday
Dinner 2: Tuesday, Thursday, and Saturday

Morning Snack 1: Monday, Wednesday, Friday, and Sunday
Morning Snack 2: Tuesday, Thursday, and Saturday

Afternoon Snack 1: Monday, Wednesday, Friday, and Sunday
Afternoon Snack 2: Tuesday, Thursday, and Saturday

Evening Snack 1: Monday, Wednesday, Friday, and Sunday
Evening Snack 2: Tuesday, Thursday, and Saturday

This plan is one of the easiest things that you can do because you will only need to buy two separate meals for each of the meals that you are eating. It is a great way to keep from getting bored while also allowing you to save money on the ingredients that you buy. Put each of your favorite recipes from the book into each slot on the meal plan and you will be good to go.

Doing this allows you the chance to truly be prepared. You will not ever be able to lose a large amount of weight if you do not plan ahead for it. Not everyone who diets uses meal plans to lose weight, but everyone who uses meal plans to diet loses weight.

You don't have to do anything complicated to plan your meals or even prep them which is a popular option in many diets. All you need to do is create a menu ahead of time and choose what you need off of it for when you go shopping for the ingredients.

Chapter 4:

Ketogenic Shopping List

Before you get started with the ketogenic diet, you will need to make sure that you have the tools to be able to complete all of the recipes that will make it easier for you to eat them... food! You will need to go shopping before you start the diet and before you are able to make the recipes so that you will get the best experience out of the diet. If you shop ahead of time for your ingredients, making them when it is time will be much easier for you because you'll have everything on-hand to help you make the recipe.

Benefits of a Shopping List

Having a shopping list that you can use will give you the chance to make sure that you are going to be able to shop easily and quickly. With the shopping list, you will need to make sure that you are buying what you need to be able to be successful at the diet. When you do this, it will give you a chance at being more successful and having an easier time making the meal plan that you are going to use.

In general, you can use the shopping list on its own or you can pick and choose what you are going to use. Obviously, not everyone is going to like everything that is on the list but you should get most the things when you are first starting out.

By keeping a very large amount of food in your home that you can eat on the ketogenic diet, it will help you make sure that you are going to be able to always have something that you can eat. If you don't have the right kind of food for your

21

diet, you may risk not being able to do the diet or use the right type of recipes.

Keep in mind that a shopping list will make it easier for you to create the meal plans and the subsequent recipes that you need to be able to do everything that will make the diet easier for you.

What About Other Family Members?

Just because you are doing the diet doesn't mean that everyone else in your house has to do it, too. Or, does it? The chances are that when you start to eat food on the ketogenic diet, everyone else will pick up the same habits that you have which will make it easier for you to do the diet.

This is especially true for "family" meals like dinner where everyone sits down and eats the same thing. If you are cooking ketogenic meals for yourself, you will also be able to cook them for your family members so that you can all eat close to the same thing while you are dieting. It is a great way for you to be able to include everyone into the healthy lifestyle that you have and with the different things that are going on in your life. Make sure that you are doing what you can to include everyone so that they can all have healthy eating habits. If you do the diet, you will be able to help your family do it, too.

If your family chooses not to do the ketogenic diet with you, make sure that you let them know that you are shopping for *your* food and if there is anything that they want that is on the "no" list, they will need to let you know before you shop or simply buy the food for themselves.

How to Avoid the "Bad" Food

Even with the best intentions and a full shopping list, your resolve can go out the window when you get to the grocery store; this is what happens to many people who are dieting. They get enticed by the advertising and pick up things that they really don't need so that they can eat them later or bring them home for someone in their family.

Don't do this. You will end up eating the food especially if it is loaded with Net carbohydrates.

To help yourself avoid the "bad" food, stay on the perimeters of the grocery store. Nearly everything that is on the "inside" of the grocery store is processed and not made for you at any time, let alone while you are doing the keto diet. You can help yourself avoid temptation by just shopping around the outside of the store, meaning vegetables, meats, and dairy are really the only things that you need.

Stay away from the pasta and chip aisles!

Make the Most of Shopping

If you are going to go to the grocery store to shop for the food that you are going to use on the diet, make sure that you get it in one sweep. Try to only go to the grocery store once per week. This will keep you from spending too much money and will also keep you from having to worry about being enticed by food that isn't going to fit in with your diet. The fewer times that you go to the store, the better chance you will have at being successful with your diet. It is a great idea to only go grocery shopping when you need to.

Some people choose to go grocery shopping when they need something. However, since you have meal plans and you know what recipes you are going to make, you don't have to worry about doing that. With the meal plans that are included and the recipes that you now have at your disposal, you can give yourself a chance to write down everything that you need before you go to the store. Start with the big master list and then, as you run out of ingredients, shop for the things that you will need for the week.

Discounts Galore!

Coupons are a great way to save money and most people use them if they want to get the best deals possible on the food that they are buying but coupons are usually only good for people who are shopping for processed foods. If you are doing the ketogenic diet, you will need to avoid most processed foods and all Net Carbohydrates so coupons might not work for you. How, though, are you supposed to get great discounts on the products that you need to help you make the best meals possible?

You're going to learn right now.

Sales!

The sales that stores have are usually on products like meat and other perishables; they may have sales on canned goods and even some dairy products depending on the time of year. You will be able to get your vegetables on sale every time that you go to the store if you know the right way to shop the sales and how to be able to provide yourself with the best opportunity possible for your food needs. It is necessary for you to shop sales. Another thing that many keto followers do is shop at discount grocers. In the past, you would have to sacrifice quality for price at these places, but that is no longer the case... most discount grocers actually have higher quality than big chains.

Customize the List

The grocery shopping list that you will be able to use at the beginning of your ketogenic diet experience is something that you can use to get everything that you need but also something that you can customize so that you can choose which options are best for you. Because of the way that you can do things with the ketogenic diet, you will be able to make sure that you are getting the best experience possible and that you are going to be able to figure out the right way to be able to get the best experience possible.

There will be some things on this list that you do not like or that you might not use during the diet. Simply don't purchase those things when you go to the store and then give yourself the opportunity to purchase *more* of what you will eat while you are doing the diet. This will help you to save time, money, and give you all the keto-friendly foods that you love.

Follow this easy shopping list before you start the diet and stock up on *all* the things that you need for keto:

- All Spice
- Almond Flour / Meal
- Almond Milk
- Anchovies
- Apples
- Apricot
- Artichokes
- Asparagus
- Avocado
- Avocado
- Baby Back Ribs
- Bacon
- Bacon Fat
- Bananas
- Bass
- Bean Sprouts
- Bell Peppers
- Béarnaise Sauce
- Blackberries
- Blue Cheese

- Blue Cheese
- Blueberries
- Bok Choy
- Brie Cheese
- Broccoli
- Brussel Sprouts
- Organic butter
- Cabbage
- Cajun Spice
- Canned Artichoke Hearts
- Canned Asparagus
- Canned Black Olives
- Canned Chicken
- Canned Green Beans
- Canned Green Olives
- Canned Greens
- Canned Mushrooms
- Canned Pickles
- Canned Salmon & Tuna
- Canned Sauerkraut
- Canned Spinach
- Capers
- Cashew Milk
- Catfish
- Cauliflower
- Celery
- Cheddar Cheese
- Cherries
- Cherry Tomatoes
- Chia Seeds
- Chicken Broth
- Chicken deli meat
- Chicken Eggs
- Chicken Legs
- Chicken Tenders
- Chicken Thighs

- ➢ Chicken Wings
- ➢ Chili Powder
- ➢ Cinnamon
- ➢ Cocoa Powder
- ➢ Coconut Flakes
- ➢ Coconut Flour
- ➢ Coconut Milk
- ➢ Coconut Oil
- ➢ Cod
- ➢ Coffee Plain
- ➢ Coffee with Cream
- ➢ Coffee without sweetener
- ➢ Colby Cheese
- ➢ Corned Beef
- ➢ Cornish Hens
- ➢ Cottage Cheese
- ➢ Crab
- ➢ Cranberries
- ➢ Cream Cheese
- ➢ Cream of Tartar
- ➢ Cucumbers
- ➢ Cumin
- ➢ Dates
- ➢ Dill
- ➢ Duck
- ➢ Duck Fat
- ➢ Eggplant
- ➢ Eggs & Meat
- ➢ Erythritol
- ➢ Feta Cheese
- ➢ Figs
- ➢ Flax Meal
- ➢ Flax Seeds
- ➢ Flounder
- ➢ Fresh Spinach
- ➢ Full Cream Greek Yogurt

- Full Cream Milk
- Full Fat Milk
- Full Fat Yogurt
- Garlic Powder
- Garlic Salt
- Goat Cheese
- Goose
- Grapefruit
- Grapes
- Green Bell Peppers
- Green Onions
- Greens
- Ground chicken
- Ground Pork
- Guava
- Haddock
- Halibut
- Ham
- Hamburger
- Heavy Whipping Cream
- Herring
- Hollandaise Sauce
- Horseradish
- Hot Peppers
- Hot Sauce
- Iceberg Lettuce
- Italian
- Keto Seafood
- Kiwi
- Leeks
- Lemon Juice
- Lemons
- Lime Juice
- Limes
- Lobster
- Low-Carb Salsa

- Mango
- Mayonnaise
- Mayonnaise
- Melons
- Monterey Jack Cheese
- Mozzarella Cheese
- Mushrooms
- Napa Cabbage
- Nectarines
- Okra
- Extra virgin olive oil
- Olives
- Onion Powder
- Orange Bell Peppers
- Orange Roughie
- Oranges
- Oregano
- Oysters
- Papaya
- Paprika
- Parmesan Cheese
- Parsley
- Passion Fruit
- Peaches
- Peanut Oil
- Pears
- Pepper
- Pheasant
- Pineapples
- Plums
- Pomegranates
- Pork Chops
- Pork Roast
- Portabella Mushrooms
- Prime Rib
- Protein Shakes

- Pumpkin Spice
- Quail
- Radishes
- Ranch
- Raspberry
- Real Bacon Bits
- Red bell peppers
- Rhubarb
- Roast Beef
- Romaine Lettuce
- Salmon
- Salt
- Sardines
- Scallops
- Sesame Oil
- Shellfish
- Shrimp
- Snow Peas
- Sole
- Sour Cream
- Soy Sauce
- Spaghetti Squash
- Spinach
- Steak
- Stevia Drops
- Strawberries
- String Cheeses
- Sugar-Free Ketchup
- Sugar-Free Syrup
- Sunflower Oil
- Swiss Cheese
- Tangerines
- Tenderloin
- Tilapia
- Tomatoes
- Trout

- Tuna Fish
- Turkey Bacon
- Turkey Breast
- Turkey deli meat
- Turkey Ground
- Turkey Legs
- Turkey Sausage
- Turmeric
- Unsweetened Tea
- Vinegar
- Whole Chicken
- Whole Turkey
- Worcestershire Sauce
- Xylitol
- Yellow and Brown Mustard
- Yellow bell peppers
- Yellow Onions
- Yellow Squash
- Zucchini

Chapter 5:

How the Ketogenic Diet Works

Now that you are aware of all the benefits of the diet and how it can help you to lose weight, you should learn more about the science behind the diet. While you already know that the diet combines the science of losing weight with the biology of the human body, there is so much more to it than just a basic understanding of the way that things can work with the body. If you want to make sure that you are doing different things with the diet and have a chance to do what you can with it, you should know what makes the diet work.

Net Carbohydrates to Glucose

When you eat carbohydrates, they are immediately converted to glucose in your body. The body then uses the glucose for energy to help you get through the process of survival. However, there are major problems with the body using glucose to be able to survive. One of the biggest issues that comes from the body using glucose is that it is:

SUGAR!

The sugar that the body takes in is not good at all. Instead of you being able to enjoy the benefits that come with eating and allowing your body to use energy, you are constantly taking in more sugar to keep up with the demands that your body is probably now accustomed to thanks to all the sugar that is present in your diet.

If you eat a lot of sugar, you will have health problems and you will not be able to lose weight. Net carbohydrates are sugar.

Why Glucose is Bad

Along with the idea that you can't lose weight if you eat Net carbohydrates because of the glucose being the main form of nutrition, you also will have other problems with your body thanks to glucose. It increases the acidity of your body and causes you to have many health problems.

Eating a lot of glucose can cause you to have tooth and gum problems, digestive issues, weight gain, memory issues, increased risk of cancer, and a higher chance of infection in your body.

Sugar wreaks havoc on the body in every way possible, and there is no way that you will ever be able to have a healthy life if your diet mainly consists of sugar and all of the things that come as a result of sugar.

Your Body – Starving

When you stop eating sugar, your body will go in to some type of shock mode. That is because it is so used to having sugar, and suddenly, there is no sugar there for it to rely on; it thinks that it is starving and that is where you want your body to be at. You don't want to *actually* starve (that would be bad, and you would die) but you do want the body to think that it is starving.

When your body believes that it is starving, it will rely on the fat that it has stored up to be able to get the nutrition that you need. Of course, simply quitting food altogether is not the way to get to this point. With the ketogenic diet, your body will be able to stay in that near-starvation mode (ketosis) while you continue to lose weight. It will help you to have a better time with the diet that you are doing and with the different options that are present in the diet. While you work to make sure that you are cutting sugar out, you will be able to take advantage of all the aspects of the diet so that you can try new things and your body will be able to go back to the way that it is supposed to be.

Back to Nature

While the ketogenic diet is quite different from the paleo diet, they do have somewhat close to the same concepts that make the diet up. The idea is that you want to be able to get the most amount of nutrition possible while you are allowing your body to go back to the way that it is supposed to be.

In nature, your body would rely on mostly vegetables and meats with some dairy in there. The same is true with the ketogenic diet. During prehistoric times, there were no grains, breads, or other processed foods for people to live off of and they were among the healthiest people that have ever been in the human race.

It is important to know that the ketogenic diet does not require you eat like a caveman, but you will help yourself out when you focus your diet around fatty dairy and meats that are rich in protein.

Energy

You will have so much more energy when you are doing the ketogenic diet, yet most people give up after only a couple of days because they *do* have reduced energy when they first cut out all those Net carbohydrates. If that is something that you are not comfortable with, consider using the approach where you can "ease" into the diet instead of just jumping in and quitting Net carbohydrates cold turkey. The energy shift that you will see once you enter ketosis is incredible and something that many people take advantage of while they are doing the diet.

What you don't realize is that Net carbohydrates, while they feel like they are fueling your body, are actually causing you to have delayed bodily reactions that will make it harder for you to get what you need out of the different aspects of your diet and the nutrition factors. If you do not do what you are supposed to with the ketogenic diet, you will find that it will be extremely difficult for you to truly get the best experience and to have what you need out of the diet.

Keep in mind that each time that you try to do the diet, you will need to make sure that you are aware of the energy benefits that come from ketosis.

Burning Fat That You Eat

When you eat a diet that is high in fat, it takes your body a very long time to convert that fat to energy. While it is able to convert it to energy and that is much healthier than the other things that you could do with other diets, it takes quite a long time, and you will need to try different things while you are doing the diet.

It is necessary for you to try and make sure that you are getting what you can out of the diet by eating as much fat as possible. While the body is trying to process the fats that you are consuming, you will need to get energy from somewhere else. This is where the fat that is stored in your body comes into play. The body will pull the fat from the "emergency" stores that it has created on your body and it will use that for energy so that it doesn't have to rely on just waiting for the fat to get done processing through the body.

Entering Ketosis

When you first start with the ketogenic diet, you will enter into what is known as ketosis. This is fat burning at its finest, and it is something that the body was designed to do to keep it from starving to death after just a few hours with no food. Ketosis can be achieved by nearly every diet but the ketogenic diet is able to bring it on much more quickly with the use of high fats and no Net carbohydrates.

Ketosis is a great place to be because it allows you to burn almost all of the fat that is on your body. As long as you are in ketosis, you will continue to burn fat and that will help you to lose the weight and the inches that you want off of your body. Since you will be doing the diet for at least a few months, ketosis will be happening throughout the entire time that you are doing the diet. It will make things easier for you to be able to get what you need out of it and it will also give you the chance to be able to try new things with your diet so that you can enjoy every aspect of it.

Checking for Ketosis

There are a few ways that you will be able to check for ketosis. The first is fairly rudimentary, and will not always be accurate. If you are sweating when you are in ketosis (which you will be, quite a bit more), your sweat will take on a different type of odor. It will be slightly sweet-smelling, and recognizable apart from what normal sweat is supposed to smell like; this is indicative that you are in the ketosis phase.

You can also check for ketosis by the smell of your urine. Urine, while you are in ketosis has a very strong and distinctive odor that you will be able to recognize. In the past, that is how people were able to tell whether or not they were in ketosis because they did not have any other way to be able to figure it out.

Now, however, there are testing strips that you can use to dip in your urine. They will test for the presence of ketones in the urine which will tell you that you are in ketosis. They can be purchased in large quantities from basic drug stores for just a few dollars per box.

Brain Health

The brain is meant to run on fatty energy. When it has been fed a steady diet of sugar, it will struggle to be able to work properly, and you may find that your hormones are not functioning the way that they should. Because of the way that the brain works and because you are able to make sure that you are doing different things *with* your brain, you will be able to benefit from the ketogenic diet.

The brain will also be better as you do the diet. Your brain is made up of many different receptors and when it realizes that you are no longer feeding it a diet that is high in sugar, it will start to recognize that and react appropriately. This is something that will help you to lose more weight and will give you a chance to see the differences that can come up in different situations. It will also help you to change the way that you do things and to make things better for your body.

While you are doing different things with your body, your brain will also be reacting.

Reduced Blood Sugar

There is no doubt that using the ketogenic diet will help to reduce your blood sugar... but what does lower blood sugar really mean for you and the way that your body is able to do different things?

Lower blood sugar will not only help you to reduce the risk that you have of diabetes, but it will also help you to have a more comfortable life. Your bones will no longer hurt; your joints won't ache and muscle stiffness will be drastically reduced if you are not dealing with high blood sugar all the time. It is important to note that high blood sugar can have very negative effects on your body, but lowered blood sugar can help it to run optimally.

When you have lower blood sugar, you will be able to reduce your risk of different things and your body will also be able to lose weight more easily. It is a great way for you to be able to try new things that you can do with your body so that you will be able to truly enjoy all the benefits that come with eating right and being as healthy as possible. Make sure that you are comfortable with the options that you have and that you can make sure that you are going to use the diet to help with blood sugar problems.

Chapter 6:

Diseases that the Ketogenic Diet Can Help

A change in your diet often is able to make a big impact on your body and the way that you are able to do things but it is not always the perfect cure all that you need for diseases. There are some diseases, though, that you can help to make better when you use the ketogenic diet.

One thing that is important to note is that you should *always* follow your doctor's advice. Just because you're doing a new diet doesn't mean that you can stop taking your medications or doing things that your doctor has told you to do. Whether you are doing the diet to help with one of your diseases, or you are simply doing it to help yourself lose weight, always take the advice of your doctor over the advice of an eBook that you downloaded online to make sure that you are as healthy as possible.

Talk to your doctor before starting any new diet plan so that you will be able to truly start out on the healthiest foot possible whether you are doing it for disease-related reasons or weight-related reasons.

Keep in mind that there is no guarantee that the ketogenic diet will help you if you have one of these diseases but there are other people who have had success with each of these diseases and the diet that has helped them to have a better chance at living a happier and healthier life.

RSD / CRPS

This disease is characterized by nerve misfires and issues that stem from other types of nerve injuries. It is painful and often debilitating to the people who have it; it does not have a cure but there are some things that can make it better.

Losing weight from the ketogenic diet, reducing sugar that the body has in it, and allowing you to have more energy are all aspects of the ketogenic diet that can help you to feel better if you have RSD or CRPS.

Be careful about the processed meats that you eat because those can sometimes cause flare-ups of the disease.

Polycystic Ovarian Syndrome

While previously thought to be a relatively rare disease, PCOS is something that is becoming more and more common. It is thought to stem from the problems that eating foods high in sugar combined with having excess weight on your body can do to the hormones. Being just 10% overweight can put you at major risk for PCOS. The good news, however, is that reducing your weight by just 10% can also help you to no longer see the symptoms that come from PCOS.

In the ketogenic diet, the idea behind ridding your body of unnecessary sugar is something that you can make yourself have a better time with and get your hormones back on the right track.

Parkinson's

There are many medications that you can take for Parkinson's, but most people who have the disease and switched to a ketogenic way of eating were able to see major improvements not only in the tremors that they had within their body but also with the different things that could happen to their body. It is not a disease that you are going to cure with diet and you should still continue to take all of your prescribed medications, but it will help you to have a more agreeable way to manage the disease.

Obesity

This is one of the only diseases that the ketogenic diet is known to cure. Because you will be losing weight with the diet and you will be doing what you can to actually lose that weight, you will be able to cure your obesity.

While obesity comes with a host of other problems, simply being able to lose the weight that is making you obese will be enough to cure those problems and to help you have a better and more enjoyable life.

MS

There are many things that you can do to help ease the symptoms of MS. While the outlook for the disease is often not good for people who have it, there are things that you can do to make it better and eating a diet that is high in protein and very low in carbohydrates is one of the best things that you can do to make yourself feel better. It will also help to reduce the inflammation that comes along with MS and the problems that it causes as a result of the inflammation.

Migraines

Migraine sufferers are constantly looking for something that will make them feel better and give them the relief that they need. The idea behind the ketogenic diet for migraines is that it will help you to reduce the negative effects that come about as a result of inflammation in the head, sinuses, and around the brain. When you use the ketogenic diet to make your migraines better, you will give yourself a better chance at being able to have a more comfortable life. Your migraines will probably not disappear completely, but the number of ones that you have will be far less than if you were eating a diet that is high in carbohydrates.

Metabolic Syndrome

Similar to diabetes, metabolic syndrome is really the last step before you have diabetes. What is commonly referred to as pre-diabetes, metabolic syndrome has a negative effect on the way that you are able to process carbohydrates and it can cause you to have blood sugar that is very high compared to what is considered "normal." If you have metabolic syndrome, you still have a chance before there is any lasting damage to your body. Turn around your life and give yourself the best chance at being able to overcome the problems that are associated with diabetes. Do not get to the point where you have diabetes.

Hidradenitis Suppurativa

What was once a rare disease is now becoming much more prevalent. Characterized by painful and embarrassing boils that crop up around the sweat glands throughout your body, Hidradenitis Suppurativa is not only uncomfortable, but also puts you at risk for dangerous infections of the blood stream.

While there is no official information on what causes HS, researchers believe that it is a result of too much sugar in the body. It is, like most other diseases, a negative response to sugar. Cutting out sugar and carbohydrates will reduce the symptoms that HS causes and can almost eliminate the symptoms completely. While it will help you to get rid of painful boils and flare ups, it will not get rid of the scars that are associated with them.

GSD

Eating a diet that has no or very few Net carbohydrates in it will help to ease the symptoms of this painful disease. While you are eating the ketogenic diet, you will be able to get the best out of it and you will also help yourself to make sure that you are not being impacted by the disease. Always check with your doctor to make sure that you are healthy enough to make a change to your diet.

Gluten Deficiency

A lack of gluten in your diet can actually help you with deficiencies that you have of gluten in your body. The artificial form of it can be harmful and will make it harder for you to process other nutrients. When you reduce the Net carbohydrates and sugar in your diet, you will also reduce the amount of gluten that you consume. It will help you to have a more enjoyable and healthy life especially if you were deficient in the past.

Fatty Liver

Since you are eating a lot of fat that is present in the diet, you would think that it wouldn't be something that could *help* the fat in your body but it actually does. Most people who are diagnosed with fatty liver disease are advised to eat a lower carbohydrate diet - the thing about eating a lot of fat is that you won't have to worry about how you are eating Net carbohydrates for fuel. Your body will function better and that will allow your liver to be able to be healthier.

Epilepsy

The ketogenic diet was originally used to help cure epilepsy. While it was not able to completely cure it, it was shown to help people who have the disease. While you should always follow your doctor's advice and take all prescribed medication for epilepsy, there are many people who have been able to stop taking anti-seizure medication just from making the switch to a more natural ketogenic diet. Carbohydrates and sugar can often bring on a seizure and trigger major problems for people who have epilepsy. Eliminating them is one step that you can take to avoid seizures.

Diabetes

Reducing obesity is just one of the ways that having a diet high in fats and proteins will help you, but actually being able to beat diabetes is one of the best diet plans in the world. If you are diagnosed with diabetes, your doctor will often give you diabetic cooking plans and recipes that you can use to make your life better and, hopefully, eliminate the diabetes that you have already gotten.

If you have just been diagnosed with diabetes, switch to a ketogenic plan that is similar to diabetic cooking options. You will be able to cure your diabetes and live a normal, healthy life.

Cancer

While there is no true cure for cancer and you may struggle with some of the problems that are associated with it, eating a diet that has little to no sugar in it will help with cancer diagnoses. You can prevent certain types of cancer by cutting out all the sugar in your diet and, if you do get cancer, you will be able to help yourself beat it using a ketogenic diet.

Keep in mind that eliminating sugar will not be able to cure all of the different types of cancer but it will be something that can help you.

Brain Injuries

Traumatic brain injuries are tricky because there are no two that are exactly alike You can help yourself with the traumatic brain injury that you have by eating a diet that is low in Net Carbohydrates. The ketogenic diet is healthy for your brain and will allow it to work less than if you were eating a diet that had a lot of Net Carbohydrates. Doing this will help your brain be better able to focus on the important things – like being able to walk and making your life better in different ways aside from the injury that you have sustained.

Autism

Parents who feed autistic children a ketogenic diet will have a much easier time with social responses and being able to help them with the cues that they need to make their lives better. Even non-speaking autistic children are able to benefit from the diet and can make sure that they are doing things the right way with the ketogenic diet. It is not hard to feed children a ketogenic diet, but do make sure that you are including some fruit and healthy sugars in the diet so that your child does not lose too much weight.

Alzheimer's

Sugar can severely damage the brain and cause it to not function in the way that it should. Because of this, you can reduce the risk for Alzheimer's disease by simply cutting out sugar. People who already have the disease and who eat a diet that is low in sugar and carbohydrates will be able to live a more comfortable life. They can reduce the symptoms that come with Alzheimer's simply by being able to eat foods that don't have Net carbohydrates in them so that they can feel better with the different things that are going on.

Part 2:

Recipes for

the

Ketogenic Diet

Chapter 7:

Breakfast Recipes

Raspberry Vanilla Yogurt

Number of Servings: 1

Time for Preparation: 15 mins

Time to Cook Recipe: 0 mins

1~ . ~cup of Greek yogurt
1~ . ~tsp of stevia
½~ . ~c raspberries

Mix up your stevia and the Greek yogurt so that they are mixed together well, then add the berries to the yogurt and serve. You can also put some mint on top for a different flavor twist.

Nutritional Facts:

Calories~ . ~177

Net Carbohydrates~ . ~4.8 g

Soluble Fat~ . ~12 g

Protein~ . ~12

Sodium~ . ~709 mg

Fiber~ . ~3 g

Healthy Blueberry Pancakes

Number of Servings: 2

Time for Preparation: 20 mins

Time to Cook Recipe: 10 mins

½ ~. ~ c almond flour

3~ . ~ cage free organic eggs

2~. ~ tbsp. coconut oil

1~. ~ tsp. vanilla

1~. ~ tbsp. coconut oil to fry

¼~. ~ c blueberries that are frozen

Combine the almond flour, eggs, and the coconut oil together until they are well mixed. Put some of the vanilla in with them and then GENTLY fold in the blueberries until they are completely combined.

When they are fully mixed, place your coconut oil in a frying pan and allow it to get hot. Pour the batter in medallions and wait until they bubble up on each side, then flip.

Nutritional Facts:

Calories~. ~208

Net Carbohydrates~. ~0 g

Soluble Fat~. ~17 g

Protein~. ~13

Sodium~. ~800 mg

Fiber~. ~12 g

Simply Perfect Quiche

Number of Servings: 4

Time for Preparation: 30 mins

Time to Cook Recipe: 20 mins

6~ . ~cage free organic eggs

2~ . ~pieces of bacon that are crumbled

¼~ . ~onion that is chopped

1~ . ~tbsp. coconut oil

1~ . ~tsp. salt

1~ . ~tsp. vegetable oil

1~ . ~tsp. thyme

1~ . ~tsp. pepper

Mix all the ingredients except for the coconut oil. Rub the inside of a pie dish with the coconut oil until it is completely coated so that the mixture does not stick to the sides of the pan.

Pour the rest of the ingredients into the pan and bake it for 20 minutes on 350 degrees. The egg should not be liquid when you take it out. Top with cheddar cheese and chives.

Nutritional Facts:

Calories~ . ~300

Net Carbohydrates~ . ~1.2 g

Soluble Fat~ . ~28 g

Protein~ . ~14

Sodium~ . ~300 mg

Fiber~ . ~12 g

Mexican Omelet

Number of Servings: 1

Time for Preparation: 15 mins

Time to Cook Recipe: 5 mins

2~. ~cage free organic eggs

1~. ~slice of bacon that is crumbled up

¼~. ~c chopped green pepper

¼~. ~c chopped onion

1~. ~tsp. chili powder

1~. ~tsp. salt

1~. ~tsp. pepper

¼~. ~c pepper jack cheese

1~. ~tbsp. organic butter

Allow the pan to heat up over the medium or medium high heat so that it gets as hot as possible. Mix up all of the ingredients in a bowl except for the organic butter to make sure that they are all blended well. The egg should be broken up in the bowl and the yolks should not be solid.

Put the organic butter into the pan and let it heat up. Pour your egg mixture into the pan and cook so that it is almost cooked the whole way through. Fold, flip, and cook for another 30 seconds. Serve hot.

Nutritional Facts:

Calories~. ~177

Net Carbohydrates~. ~4.8 g

Soluble Fat~. ~12 g

Protein~. ~12

Sodium~. ~709 mg

Fiber~. ~3 g

Fluffy Cakes

Number of Servings: 3

Time for Preparation: 20 mins

Time to Cook Recipe: 10 mins

½~. ~c cream cheese

2~. ~cage free organic eggs

2~. ~tsp. stevia

1~. ~tbsp. coconut oil

Be sure that the cream cheese is as soft as possible (but not melted) so that it will be easier for you to work with. Heat the coconut oil in a cast iron skillet until it starts to get very hot and bubbles up. Blend the eggs and the cream cheese together and add in the stevia so that the pancakes have a traditional flavor. For savory pancakes, leave the stevia out. Pour the ingredients into the pan and allow it to bubble up. Only flip when it is completely bubbling. Serve hot.

Coconut Yogurt

Number of Servings: 1

Time for Preparation: 5 mins

Time to Cook Recipe: 0 minx

1~. ~c Greek yogurt, plain

1~. ~tsp. coconut extract

1~. ~tsp. shredded coconut

6~. ~raspberries

Combine the extract with the yogurt and stir it so that it is mixed together well. Add more for a stronger flavor. Put in a ramekin and top with the shredded coconut and the raspberries. The raspberries can be detrimental to the diet, so make sure that you only eat six or fewer.

Nutritional Facts:

Calories~. ~154

Net Carbohydrates~. ~.2 g

Soluble Fat~. ~8 g

Protein~. ~16

Sodium~. ~688 mg

Fiber~. ~10 g

"Cereal"

Number of Servings: 1

Time for Preparation: 10 mins

Time to Cook Recipe: 0 mins

½~. ~c coconut flakes that are unsweetened

¾~. ~c coconut milk

1~. ~tsp stevia

Combine all of the ingredients together and make sure that they are all mixed up so that they are like a porridge or cold cereal. You can top with cinnamon for an interesting twist, or sprinkle with a small amount of ginger for a zing that will help you to get going in the morning with the cereal that you eat.

Nutritional Facts:

Calories~. ~138

Net Carbohydrates~. ~2.1 g

Soluble Fat~. ~13 g

Protein~. ~5

Sodium~. ~309 mg

Fiber~. ~5 g

Yogurt with Spices

Number of Servings: 1

Time for Preparation: 5 mins

Time to Cook Recipe: 0 mins

1~. ~c plain Greek yogurt

1~. ~tsp. stevia

1~. ~tsp. maple extract (NOT maple syrup)

1~. ~tbsp. walnuts

Chop walnuts up in a food processor, or simply purchase them so that they are chopped up already when you start the recipe. Make sure that you mix the yogurt and the maple extract first so that the flavors will be able to combine together. You can also use some vanilla extract in addition to the maple. Once that is mixed up the whole way, mix the stevia in with the yogurt. Top with walnuts and serve. Do not eat more than 1 tbsp. of walnuts as they are filled with Net carbohydrates.

Nutritional Facts:

Calories~. ~177

Net Carbohydrates~. ~4.8 g

Soluble Fat~. ~12 g

Protein~. ~12

Sodium~. ~709 mg

Fiber~. ~3 g

Flaxseed Hotcakes

Number of Servings: 1

Time for Preparation: 15 mins

Time to Cook Recipe: 5 mins

½~. ~c cream cheese

2~. ~cage free organic eggs

2~. ~tbsp. crushed flaxseed

2~. ~tsp. stevia

1~. ~tbsp. coconut oil

Lay your cream cheese out ahead of time so that it will be soft by the time that you do this recipe. Use a hand mixer and beat the cream cheese with the eggs and the stevia. Slowly add in the crushed flaxseed, and mix it so that it is like a batter with the other ingredients. Put a pan on the stove and heat it up so that it is on medium or high heat. Put the coconut oil in and give it a chance to be able to melt. Drop a spoonful of the hotcake batter into the coconut oil and cook until fully done so that the hotcakes will be fully cooked both inside and outside. Make sure that you are cooking them enough on each side. Serve them so that they are still hot. Top with a dollop of heavy whipping cream for additional flavor, or add some chives to give them the savory taste.

Calories~. ~214

Net Carbohydrates~. ~4 g

Fat ~19 g

Protein~. ~8 g

Sodium~. ~380 mg

Fiber~. ~1 g

Colorful Peppery Casserole

Number of Servings: 4

Time for Preparation: 15 minutes

Time to Cook Recipe: 30 mins

Ingredients:

½~. ~red bell pepper~. ~diced

½~. ~green bell pepper~. ~diced

½~. ~yellow bell pepper~. ~diced

½ c~. ~almond dairy milk

One can~. ~artichoke hearts~. ~drained

8~. ~cage free organic eggs

One tsp~. ~oregano

1 tsp. .~. ~black pepper

1 tsp. .~. ~salt

1 splash~. ~olive oil

Put all of your ingredients into a pan that has been greased with extra virgin olive oil.

Cook on 350 degrees for 35 minutes.

Nutritional Facts:

Calories~. ~177

Net Carbohydrates~. ~4.8 g

Soluble Fat~. ~12 g

Protein~. ~12

Sodium~. ~709 mg

Fiber~. ~3 g

Not Oatmeal

Number of Servings: 5

Time for Preparation: 15 minutes

Time to Cook Recipe: 15 mins

Ingredients:

¼ c~. ~flaxseed

¼ c~. ~almonds~. ~chopped

¼ c~. ~walnuts~. ~chopped

1 c~. ~coconut milk

1 c~. ~cold water

1 tsp. .~. ~almond organic butter

1 tsp. .~. ~cardamom

1 tsp. .~. ~ghee or organic butter

Put all of the ingredients that you have into a large sauce pan and mix them up so that they are well combined.

Cook for 15 minutes, stirring often so that it does not burn.

Nutritional Facts:

Calories~. ~266

Net Carbohydrates~. ~5.2 g

Soluble Fat~. ~20 g

Protein~. ~5 g

Sodium~. ~9 mg

Fiber~. ~2 g

Bagel of Meat

Number of Servings: 3

Time for Preparation: 15 minutes

Time to Cook Recipe: 30 mins

Ingredients:

1 lb~. ~ground beef~. ~not reduced fat

1 tbsp.~. ~almond flour

1 tbsp.~. ~black pepper

2 tbsp.~. ~coconut milk

1 tsp. .~. ~salt

Splash~. ~olive oil

3 slices~. ~cheddar

1~. ~tomato~. ~sliced

1 c~. ~lettuce~. ~chopped

Form your meat into a ball and mix with the rest of the ingredients. Use your hands to make a bagel shape out of it and then fry it in a cast iron skillet until it is cooked the whole way. Top with tomato and cheese and allow it to melt.

Nutritional Facts:

Calories~. ~499

Net Carbohydrates~. ~5 g

Soluble Fat~. ~28 g

Protein~. ~55

Sodium~. ~1055 mg

Fiber~. ~1 g

Texas Breakfast

Number of Servings: 6

Time for Preparation: 20 mins

Time to Cook Recipe: 20 mins

Ingredients:

½~. ~green bell pepper~. ~diced

8~. ~cage free organic eggs

½~. ~tomato~. ~diced

1 package~. ~ranch dressing mix

1 small can~. ~black olives – drained

½ can~. ~corn~. ~drained

½ can~. ~chiles~. ~drained

1 tbsp.~. ~garlic~. ~minced

1 c~. ~pepper jack cheese~. ~shredded and divided

1 splash~. ~olive oil

Rub extra virgin olive oil all over a baking dish. Mix the rest of the ingredients into a large bowl so that they are all completely combined together. Pour them in the baking dish and put them in the oven at 400 degrees for 20 minutes.

Nutritional Facts:

Calories~. ~383

Net Carbohydrates~. ~2.1 g

Soluble Fat~. ~16 g

Protein~. ~29

Sodium~. ~677 mg

Fiber~. ~2 g

Quiche with Ham and Zucchini

Number of Servings: 4

Time for Preparation: 15 minutes

Time to Cook Recipe: 20 mins

Ingredients:

2~. ~zucchini~. ~peeled and sliced

1 lb~. ~deli meat ham~. ~chipped

12~. ~cage free organic eggs

1 tsp. .~. ~salt

1 tsp. .~. ~pepper

splash~. ~olive oil

Rub down a pie dish with extra virgin olive oil to keep it from sticking. Lay the zucchini on the bottom of the pan and cover with ham. Mix the eggs with the salt and pepper and then pour over top of it. Cook for 20 mins on 350 degrees.

Nutritional Facts:

Calories~. ~278

Net Carbohydrates~. ~2.4 g

Soluble Fat~. ~18 g

Protein~. ~5 g

Sodium~. ~605 mg

Fiber~. ~2 g

Sausage Strata

Number of Servings: 4

Time for Preparation: 15 minutes

Time to Cook Recipe: 4 hours

Ingredients:

20~. ~crimini mushrooms

2 links~. ~Italian sausage

½ c~. ~mozzarella~. ~shredded

2 tbsp.~. ~heavy cream

¼ c~. ~chicken stock

1 tsp. .~. ~oregano

2 tsp.~. ~salt

1 tsp. .~. ~black pepper

2 tbsp.~. ~organic butter

splash~. ~olive oil

Put extra virgin olive oil into the bottom of a slow cooker. Add all of the rest of the ingredients to the cooker and then put the lid on. Cook it on the high setting for 4 hours, or until the sausage is cooked through. You can also put it on the low setting and allow it to cook overnight.

Nutritional Facts:

Calories~. ~240

Net Carbohydrates~. ~4.9 g

Soluble Fat~. ~10 g

Protein~. ~8 g

Sodium~. ~1300 mg

Fiber~. ~2 g

Greens Quiche

Number of Servings: 4

Time for Preparation: 15 minutes

Time to Cook Recipe: 20 mins

Ingredients:

8~. ~cage free organic eggs

1 c~. ~spinach~. ~chopped

1 tbsp.~. ~coconut flour

¾ c~. ~walnuts~. ~chopped

1/3 c~. ~sunflower seeds~. ~shelled

1~. ~onion~. ~diced

¼ c~. ~organic butter~. ~cold

½ c~. ~mozzarella~. ~shredded

½ tsp.~. ~black pepper

1 tsp. .~. ~salt

splash~. ~olive oil

Rub your extra virgin olive oil onto the bottom of a baking dish or a pie dish. Mix the rest of the ingredients well and then pour them into the dish. Cook on 400 degrees for 20 minutes.

Nutritional Facts:

Calories~. ~298

Net Carbohydrates~. ~5.6 g

Soluble Fat~. ~22 g

Protein~. ~19

Sodium~. ~418 mg

Fiber~. ~2 g

Chapter 8:

Lunch Recipes

No Guilt Spinach Dip

Number of Servings: 6

Time for Preparation: 20 minutes

Time to Cook Recipe: 10 minutes

Ingredients:

6 c~. ~spinach~. ~chopped

½ c~. ~canned artichoke hearts

½ c~. ~cream cheese

½ c~. ~asiago cheese~. ~grated

½ c~. ~almond dairy milk

1 tsp. .~. ~black pepper

splash~. ~olive oil

Make sure that the cream cheese is softened before you start the recipe. When you have done that, use a blender to combine the ingredients except for the asiago and the artichoke hearts. When it is completely combined, mix in the artichoke hearts. Cook for 10 minutes on low heat and allow everything to get mixed up together. Top with asiago.

Nutritional Facts:

Calories~. ~214

Net Carbohydrates~. ~4 g

Fat ~19 g

Protein~. ~8 g

Sodium~. ~380 mg

Fiber~. ~1 g

Curry Chicken Sampler

Number of Servings: 4

Time for Preparation: 10 minutes

Time to Cook Recipe: 30 minutes

Ingredients:

1 lb~. ~breast of chicken~. ~no skin or bones

4 cloves~. ~garlic~. ~grated

2 c~. ~chicken stock

1 tsp. .~. ~ginger~. ~grated

2~. ~juiced lemons

1 tsp. .~. ~coriander or cilantro

1 tsp. .~. ~cumin

½ tsp.~. ~fenugreek

1 tbsp.~. ~curry powder

½ tsp.~. ~cinnamon

1 tsp. .~. ~black pepper

1 tsp. .~. ~salt

1 splash~. ~olive oil

Cook the chicken through so that it is completely done. You can do this on a grill or using some other type of cooking method. Then, mix all of the ingredients together into a large sauce pan. Put the heat on medium or medium-high and cover it. Allow it to cook for 30 minutes, or until it is completely done.

Nutritional Facts:

Calories~. ~234

Net Carbohydrates~. ~3 g

Soluble Fat~. ~8 g

Protein~. ~38 g

Sodium~. ~782 mg

Fiber~. ~0 g

Spiced Up Jicama Wedges

Number of Servings: 8

Time for Preparation: 35 minutes

Time to Cook Recipe: 1 hour

Ingredients:

1 lb~. ~jicama~. ~peeled

1 tsp. .~. ~paprika

½ tsp.~. ~parsley

1 tsp. .~. ~black pepper

1 tsp. .~. ~salt

1 splash~. ~olive oil

1 tsp. .~. ~dill~. ~chopped

¼ c~. ~cilantro

½ tsp.~. ~salt

1 tsp. .~. ~paprika

1 tsp. .~. ~pepper

2~. ~juiced lemons

¼ c~. ~olive oil

Coat the jicama with salt, pepper, parsley, and paprika. Put the jicama on a pan that has been lined with foil and cook for 10 minutes at 350 degrees. Take them out of the oven, flip them, and cook for another 10 minutes or until they are completely done.

Combined the last 7 ingredients together and put them in the fridge while the jicama is cooking.

Dip your jicama in the mixture that you made all together.

Nutritional Facts:

Calories~. ~94

Net Carbohydrates~. ~5.2 g

Soluble Fat~. ~8 g

Protein~. ~1 g

Sodium~. ~879 mg

Fiber~. ~1 g

Wings – Asian Style

Number of Servings: 4

Time for Preparation: 10 minutes

Time to Cook Recipe: 1 hour

Ingredients:

2 lb~. ~chicken wings

2 tsp.~. ~ginger~. ~grated

2 tbsp.~. ~garlic~. ~minced

¼ c~. ~soy sauce

1 splash~. ~sesame

Mix all of the ingredients together so that they are well combined and the wings are coated. Put the wings on the grill for about 10 minutes over 500 degree heat. When they are crispy on the outside, transfer to a pan and allow them to cook on   for about 40 minutes or until they are completely done on the inside.

Nutritional Facts (4 wings):

Calories~. ~354

Net Carbohydrates~. ~5.5 g

Soluble Fat~. ~16 g

Protein~. ~45 g

Sodium~. ~730 mg

Fiber~. ~0 g

Pizza Mushrooms

Number of Servings: 8

Time for Preparation: 15 minutes

Time to Cook Recipe: 20 mins

Ingredients:

8~. ~portabella mushrooms

½ lb~. ~ground beef

1 medium~. ~onion~. ~diced

1 tbsp.~. ~garlic~. ~minced

½ c~. ~mozzarella~. ~shredded

1 large can~. ~crushed tomatoes

¼ c~. ~parmesan~. ~grated

½ tsp.~. ~oregano

1 tsp. .~. ~salt

1 tsp. .~. ~black pepper

1 tbsp.~. ~olive oil

Put tin foil around a baking pan and lay out the mushrooms so that the open part is on top.

Cook your ground beef with your onion and yourgarlic so that it is fully cooked the whole way through. Put all of the ingredients into the bottoms of the mushrooms. Set your oven to 350 degrees and allow the mushrooms to cook for 20 minutes or until the cheese is melted.

Nutritional Facts:

Calories~. ~106

Net Carbohydrates~. ~5.6 g

Soluble Fat~. ~3 g

Protein ~13 g

Sodium~. ~421 mg

Fiber~. ~2 g

Low-carb BLT Dip

Number of Servings: 6

Time for Preparation: 15 minutes

Time to Cook Recipe: 30 mins

Ingredients:

1~. ~box of cream cheese~. ~softened

1 lb~. ~cooked bacon~. ~crumbled

1 can~. ~tomatoes~. ~diced

2 c~. ~mayonnaise

1 tsp. .~. ~salt

1 tsp. ~. ~pepper

3 c~. ~lettuce~. ~chopped

1 c~. ~cheddar cheese

Put all of the ingredient,s except lettuce, in a large sauce pan and allow it to heat up over low heat. Do not let it boil, but cook it for about 30 minutes, stirring often. When it is done, take it off of the heat and fold the chopped lettuce into it. You can put additional cheddar cheese on top after the dip is done cooking.

Nutritional Facts:

Calories~. ~124

Net Carbohydrates~. ~1.1 g

Soluble Fat~. ~18 g

Protein~. ~3 g

Sodium~. ~1523 mg

Fiber~. ~5 g

Flavors of Fall Soup

Number of Servings: 8

Time for Preparation: 15 minutes

Time to Cook Recipe: 5 hours

Ingredients:

1~. ~acorn squash

1~. ~yellow bell pepper~. ~diced

2~. ~carrots~. ~sliced small

1~. ~onion~. ~diced

2 tbsp.~. ~ginger~. ~grated

1 c~. ~coconut milk

2 c~. ~chicken broth

1 tsp. ~. ~paprika

1 tsp. ~. ~salt

1 splash~. ~olive oil

Put all of your ingredients into a slow cooker. Put the lid on, and cook on low for 5 hours. When it is done, top with a bit of shredded asiago cheese.

Alternatively, you can put all of the ingredients into a large stock pot and cook on low for 1 hour.

Nutritional Facts:

Calories~. ~140

Net Carbohydrates~. ~8 g

Soluble Fat~. ~12 g

Protein~. ~2 g

Sodium~. ~315 mg

Fiber~. ~1 g

Leftover Thanksgiving Soup

Number of Servings: 8

Time for Preparation: 15 minutes

Time to Cook Recipe: 1

Ingredients:

2 ½ lbs~. ~turkey breast that is cooked

6 c~. ~spinach~. ~chopped

1~. ~onion~. ~diced

4 cloves~. ~garlic~. ~minced

2 c~. ~chicken stock

1 tsp. ~. ~rosemary

½ tsp.~. ~thyme

1 tsp. ~. ~salt

1 tsp. ~. ~pepper

1 splash~. ~olive oil

Once the turkey breast is cooked the whole way through, cut it up so that it is in small cubes and diced into pieces. Put all of the ingredients into a large sauce pan and heat it up over low or low-medium heat until it is cooked and very hot. Do not let it come to a boil and stir often to keep it from burning. Serve hot.

Nutritional Facts:

Calories~. ~193

Net Carbohydrates~. ~8.8 g

Soluble Fat~. ~6 g

Protein~. ~25 g

Sodium~. ~1780 mg

Fiber~. ~0 g

Keto Chili

Number of Servings: 6

Time for Preparation: 15 minutes

Time to Cook Recipe: 7 hours

Ingredients:

1 lb~. ~chicken that is ground

2~. ~tomatoes~. ~chopped

1~. ~green bell pepper~. ~seeded and diced

1~. ~onion that is medium

4 cloves~. ~garlic~. ~minced

2 tbsp.~. ~tomato paste

1 tsp. ~. ~oregano

1 tsp. ~. ~cumin

1 tsp. ~. ~salt

1 tsp. ~. ~black pepper

splash~. ~olive oil

Cook your ground chicken with the pepper and the onion so that it takes on the flavor. Mix the garlic in and then transfer everything to a slow cooker. Mix all of the ingredients up inside of the cooking part of the slow cooker and set it to low for 7 hours.

Nutritional Facts:

Calories~. ~161

Net Carbohydrates~. ~5 g

Soluble Fat~. ~8 g

Protein~. ~17

Sodium~. ~346 mg

Fiber~. ~2 g

Cheesy Broccoli Soup

Number of Servings: 8

Time for Preparation: 10 minutes

Time to Cook Recipe: 1 hour

Ingredients:

3 c~. ~broccoli that has been cut into bite sized pieces

½ c~. ~cashews~. ~chopped

½ c~. ~cheddar cheese~. ~shredded

2 c~. ~chicken stock

1 c~. ~coconut milk

1 tsp. ~. ~coconut flour

1 tsp. ~. ~salt

1 tsp. ~. ~black pepper

splash~. ~olive oil

¼ c~. ~organic butter

Mix all of the ingredients together in a large sauce pan. Cook it over low heat until it starts to boil but do not let it come to a full boil. When it is done cooking, you can put an immersion blender into the hot soup to let all of the flavors combine. If you want to use a different blender, simply wait until it has cooled down and transfer it to a more traditional blender.

Nutritional Facts:

Calories~. ~216

Net Carbohydrates~. ~7 g

Soluble Fat~. ~20 g

Protein ~5 g

Sodium~. ~386 mg

Fiber~. ~0 g

Skinny Soup

Number of Servings: 10

Time for Preparation: 15 minutes

Time to Cook Recipe: 1 hour

Ingredients:

½~. ~red bell pepper~. ~diced

1 can~. ~diced tomatoes

1 box~. ~chicken broth

1 head~. ~cabbage~. ~chopped small

1 can~. ~corn~. ~drained

1 can~. ~green beans~. ~drained

5 stalks~. ~celery~. ~chopped

6~. ~carrots~. ~chopped

1 tsp. ~. ~oregano

1 tsp. ~. ~black pepper

1 tsp. ~. ~salt

1 splash~. ~olive oil

Mix all of your ingredients together and put them into a stock pot. Put the pot on medium heat and allow it to cook for one hour. You should only cook long enough to soften the ingredients and allow them to have the flavors combined with each other.

Nutritional Facts:

Calories~. ~177

Net Carbohydrates~. ~4.8 g

Soluble Fat~. ~12 g

Protein~. ~12

Sodium~. ~709 mg

Fiber~. ~3 g

Bacon Wrap

Number of Servings: 2

Time for Preparation: 5 minutes

Time to Cook Recipe: 0 minutes

4~. ~leaves romaine

4~. ~pieces of cooked bacon

1~. ~c spinach

1~. ~avocado

Once the bacon is cooked the whole way, lay your lettuce leaves out on the counter that is clean. Divide the avocado into four pieces and gently rub the avocado onto the lettuce. Place the bacon on top of that and then divide the spinach into four parts and put some on each of the pieces of lettuce with bacon. Roll the lettuce up (similar to a burrito) and then put a tooth pick in it to help stabilize it.

Nutritional Facts:

Calories~. ~150

Net Carbohydrates~. ~1.2 g

Soluble Fat~. ~16 g

Protein~. ~8

Sodium~. ~500 mg

Fiber~. ~6 g

Burger for Lunch

Number of Servings: 1

Time for Preparation: 6 minutes

Time to Cook Recipe: 10 minutes

1~. ~beef patty, not lean

1~. ~tsp coconut oil

1~. ~c greens

½~. ~avocado, ripe

1~. ~tbsp. extra virgin olive oil

1~. ~tsp salt

1~. ~tsp pepper

Use the medium or the medium to high function on your stove and then put a cast iron skillet on the stove so that it will be able to heat up. Put some of the coconut oil into the pan and heat it up. Place the burger into it. Cook the burger the whole way, it should take about 10 minutes.

When it is done, take it out and cut up all of the ingredients so that they are about the same size. Toss together in a large salad bowl and then drizzle with extra virgin olive oil, salt and pepper so that it will be able to get mixed together and have the "salad" and the burger combined.

Pickle-y Egg Salad

Number of Servings: 1

Time for preparation: 10 minutes

Time to Cook Recipe: 8 minutes

2~. ~cage free organic eggs

1~. ~tbsp. mayonnaise

1~. ~tsp salt

1~. ~tsp pepper

½~. ~tsp dill, dried

1~. ~stalk of celery

1~. ~c spinach

Boil wat in a relatively small sauce pan. Put your eggs into it and then allow them to cook for about eight minutes. Take them out of the pan and allow them to cool off for a few minutes. Take the shells off of them and put them in a large bowl so that you can chop them up. Cut the celery so that it is very fine. Mix all of the ingredients except for the spinach together so that it forms a salad. Lay the spinach out on a plate or serving dish and top with the egg salad. Serve immediately.

Nutritional Facts:

Calories~. ~208

Net Carbohydrates~. ~3.8 g

Soluble Fat~. ~18 g

Protein~. ~20

Sodium~. ~189 mg

Fiber~. ~3 g

Keto Cobb Salad

Number of Servings: 1

Time for Preparation: 10 minutes

Time to Cook Recipe: 10 minutes

1~. ~organic chicken breast that has been cooked the whole way

1~. ~piece of bacon that is cooked

2~. ~c lettuce

½~. ~avocado

3~. ~cherry tomatoes

¼~. ~sliced English cucumber

1~. ~tbsp. extra virgin olive oil

1~. ~boiled egg that is diced

Make sure that all of the ingredients are rinsed and dried really well. Cut up the bacon, the organic chicken breast and the lettuce so that they are all about the same size. Cut up the avocado and the cherry tomatoes in half. Once you have sliced the cucumber, mix all of the ingredients together. You can use Italian dressing on the salad that does not have Net Carbohydrates or you can sprinkle extra virgin olive oil and vinegar on top of the salad.

Nutritional Facts:

Calories~. ~143

Net Carbohydrates~. ~2.5 g

Soluble Fat~. ~12 g

Protein~. ~10

Sodium~. ~456 mg

Fiber~. ~9 g

Flavorful Cauliflower Soup

Number of Servings: 4

Time for Preparation: 10 minutes

Time to Cook Recipe: 12 minutes

1~. ~c heavy cream

½~. ~lb bacon

3~. ~c chicken stock

2~. ~c cauliflower, chopped

1~. ~tsp salt

1~. ~tsp pepper

1~. ~tsp thyme

Cook the bacon in a pan and save the fat from the bacon. Make sure that you crumble the bacon once it has cooled down some. Mix all of the ingredients together into a large sauce pan and include the bacon grease that you saved in the pan. Cook on high for about 12 minutes so that it is cooked the whole way through. When it is done, use an immersion blender to further break up the pieces of cauliflower.

Nutritional Facts:

Calories~. ~189

Net Carbohydrates~. ~2 g

Soluble Fat~. ~6 g

Protein~. ~14

Sodium~. ~893 mg

Fiber~. ~7 g

Curry Salad

Number of Servings: 1

Time for Preparation: 10 minutes

Time to Cook Recipe: 10 minutes

1~. ~organic chicken breast

1~. ~tbsp. coconut oil

3~. ~tbsp. cream cheese

1~. ~tsp chili powder

1~. ~tsp coriander

1~. ~tsp garlic powder

1~. ~tsp onion powder

Mix the cream cheese with the coconut oil in a stand mixer. Put the rest of the ingredients except for the chicken to the cream cheese and blend it well. Cook the chicken your favorite way, grilled tastes very good with this recipe. Shred the chicken up and then mix it together with the cream cheese mixture. Serve on a bed of lettuce.

Nutritional Facts:

Calories~. ~308

Net Carbohydrates~. ~0 g

Soluble Fat~. ~15 g

Protein~. ~8

Sodium~. ~1206 mg

Fiber~. ~5 g

Carbless Bread

Number of Servings: 8

Time for Preparation: 5 minutes

Time to Cook Recipe: 3 minutes

1~. ~8 oz block of cream cheese that is soft

4~. ~cage free organic eggs

1~. ~pinch of salt

Heat your oven so that it is 350 degrees. Lay parchment paper on a baking sheet. use a mixer to combine the eggs, the salt and the cream cheese so that they are well blended together. You do not need to whip it. When it is fully combined, put it in dollops on the baking sheet that you just laid out. Put in the oven for about 3 minutes or until it starts to puff up. Take it out and let it cool down and then serve as bread.

Nutritional Facts:

Calories~. ~100

Net Carbohydrates~. ~0 g

Soluble Fat~. ~9 g

Protein~. ~15

Sodium~. ~203 mg

Fiber~. ~0 g

Cauliflower Rice

Number of Servings: 6

Time for Preparation: 5 minutes

Time to Cook Recipe: 15 minutes

1~. ~cauliflower head

Cut the cauliflower so that it is just the florets and the stalk is gone. Put the florets into a food processor and then pulse it for one minute. It will take on the appearance of rice with small pieces. Do not pulse any further after that.

Put it on a baking sheet and spread it out so that it is all in one layer.

Bake it for about 8 minutes. Take it out of the oven, use a spoon or oven mitt to spread it around even more and mix it up. Put it back in for another 7 minutes.

Nutritional Facts:

Calories~. ~89

Net Carbohydrates~. ~0 g

Soluble Fat~. ~0 g

Protein~. ~1

Sodium~. ~0 mg

Fiber~. ~8 g

Mashed Not Potatoes

Number of Servings: 6

Time for Preparation: 5 minutes

Time to Cook Recipe: 10 minutes

3~. ~c cauliflower florets

6~. ~tbsp. organic butter

4~. ~tbsp. parmesan that is grated

2~. ~tbsp. sour cream

2~. ~tbsp. cream cheese

2~. ~tbsp. heavy cream

1~. ~tsp garlic, minced

1~. ~tsp salt

½~. ~tsp pepper

Fill a large stock pot with water and cook the cauliflower until it is soft. Lay the rest of the ingredients out to soften them. Drain the cauliflower and put it into a food process. Put the rest of the ingredients into the processor and allow it to blend for about 1 minute. It should be smooth and look like mashed potatoes. Top with additional sour cream and green onion that is chopped.

Nutritional Facts:

Calories ~403

Net Carbohydrates~. ~2 g

Soluble Fat~. ~16 g

Protein~. ~4

Sodium~. ~900 mg

Fiber~. ~10 g

Pizza No Carb

Number of Servings: 4

Time for Preparation: 10 minutes

Time to Cook Recipe: 25 minutes

1 ½~. ~c mozzarella

½~. ~c cheddar

1~. ~egg

½~. ~tsp pepper

¼~. ~tsp salt

¼~. ~c sugar free pizza sauce

20~. ~slices of pepperoni

Set the oven to 450. Mix up the mozzarella and the cheddar. Stir in the egg and the seasonings so that it is fully mixed together. It will look like a ball of dough when you have it completely mixed up. Use a pizza pan, line with parchment paper and spread the cheese mixture out so that you will be able to make a crust-like formation. Put it in the oven for 15 minutes. It will be a golden color, take it out of the oven, put the sauce, extra cheese and pepperoni. Cook for 10 more minutes.

Nutritional Facts:

Calories~. ~502

Net Carbohydrates~. ~0 g

Soluble Fat~. ~19 g

Protein~. ~13

Sodium~. ~1204 mg

Fiber~. ~0 g

"Noodles"

Number of Servings: 8

Time for Preparation: 30 minutes

Time to Cook Recipe: 90 minutes

1~. ~large spaghetti squash

Poke a lot of holes all around the squash. Put it on a baking pan and put it in a preheated 350 degree oven. Cook it for 1 ½ hour. When it is done cooking, take it out and cool it down so that you can cut it open. Cut it lengthwise and then scrape the insides with a fork. The flesh will resemble noodles.

Nutritional Facts:

Calories~. ~70

Net Carbohydrates~. ~0 g

Soluble Fat~. ~0 g

Protein~. ~0

Sodium~. ~0 mg

Fiber~. ~8 g

Almond Bread

Number of Servings: 12

Time for Preparation: 15 minutes

Time to Cook Recipe: 40 minutes

½~. ~c whey protein

1/8~. ~tsp salt

2~. ~tsp baking powder

½~. ~c almond organic butter

4~. ~cage free organic eggs

1~. ~tbsp. organic butter

Use the organic butter to rub a bread pan. Put the oven on 300 degrees. Mix all of the ingredients so that they are well combined and dough-like in texture. Put the dough into the bread loaf pan and bake for about 40 minutes. It will be firm and a knife will come out clean. Run your knife around the outside, flip upside down and allow to fall on a cooling rack. Slice. Cover with plastic food wrap.

Nutritional Facts:

Calories~. ~177

Net Carbohydrates~. ~4.8 g

Soluble Fat~. ~12 g

Protein~. ~12

Sodium~. ~709 mg

Fiber~. ~3 g

Chapter 9:

Dinner Recipes

Skinny Lasagna

Number of Servings: 9

Time for Preparation: 20 minutes

Time to Cook Recipe: 60 minutes

2~. ~tbsp. extra virgin olive oil

1~. ~c onion, chopped

1~. ~tsp garlic that is minced

1~. ~lb ground beef, cooked

2~. ~tbsp. oregano

¼~. ~tsp salt

1~. ~tbsp. basil

2~. ~zucchiuni sliced lengthwise

1~. ~c ricotta cheese

2~. ~c mozzarella

¼~. ~c parmesan

¼~. ~tsp pepper

Heat your oven up to 60 degrees. Lay the zucchini out and mix the ground beef with the rest of the ingredients. Put the zucchini in the bottom of the pan, top with ground beef and cheese, then use more zucchini. Do this until you are out of zucchini finishing with cheese on top. Bake for 60 minutes or until the cheese is bubbly.

Nutritional Facts:

Calories~. ~295

Net Carbohydrates~. ~2 g

Soluble Fat~. ~13 g

Protein~. ~19

Sodium~. ~500 mg

Fiber~. ~6 g

Mexican Lime Chicken

Number of Servings: 4

Time for Preparation: 10 minutes

Time to Cook Recipe: 40 minutes

8~. ~chicken thighs~. ~skinless boneless

2 c~. ~savoy cabbage~. ~chopped

1~. ~celery~. ~diced

1~. ~onion~. ~diced

1 tbsp~. ~ginger~. ~grated

2~. ~limes

1 tsp. ~. ~salt

1 tsp. ~. ~pepper

splash~. ~olive oil

Rub extra virgin olive oil into the bottom of a large pot. Put the chicken in the bottom of it. Follow with the celery, the onion and the seasoning including the lime juice so that you can make sure that it is going to pick up those flavors. Put the cabbage on top of it and put a lid on it. Allow it to cook for about 30 minutes, stirring every 10 minutes or so. Serve hot.

Nutritional Facts:

Calories~. ~273

Net Carbohydrates~. ~5.7 g

Soluble Fat~. ~12 g

Protein~. ~34 g

Sodium~. ~689 mg

Fiber~. ~6 g

Lamb Casserole

Number of Servings: 6

Time for Preparation: 20 minutes

Time to Cook Recipe: 1 hour

4~. ~zucchini~. ~peeled

1 lb~. ~ground lamb

½ c~. ~coconut milk

2~. ~cage free organic eggs

¼ c~. ~parmesan cheese~. ~grated

½ tsp~. ~cinnamon

½ tsp~. ~cloves

½ tsp~. ~cumin

1 tsp. ~. ~garam masala

1 tsp. ~salt

1 tsp. ~. ~pepper

splash~. ~olive oil

Layer the zucchini that has been cut into long slices on the bottom of a casserole dish. Cook the lamb with the rest of the ingredients so that it is able to pick up the flavors. Make sure that it is fully cooked. Layer it on top of the zucchini then put more zucchini. Do this while you are adding more ingredients to it and make sure that you end with meat.

Nutritional Facts:

Calories~. ~403

Net Carbohydrates~. ~4.7 g

Soluble Fat~. ~10 g

Protein~. ~25 g

Sodium~. ~479 mg

Fiber~. ~3 g

Asian Beef and Broccoli

Number of Servings: 4

Time for Preparation: 10 minutes

Time to Cook Recipe: 4 hours

1 lb~. ~steak, sirloin

3 c~. ~frozen broccoli

1 c~. ~beef stock

1 tbsp~. ~ginger~. ~grated

½ tsp~. ~thyme

1 tsp. ~. ~salt

1 tsp. ~. ~pepper

splash~. ~olive oil

Slice the steak into 1-inch wide strips. Toss all of the ingredients together into a large slow cooker and make sure that it is all mixed up well so that the flavors can come together. Put the lid on the slow cooker and cook for 4 hours on high. To give yourself more time to cook, you can also cook for 8 hours on low.

Nutritional Facts:

Calories~. ~357

Net Carbohydrates~. ~6 g

Soluble Fat~. ~11 g

Protein~. ~37 g

Sodium~. ~714 mg

Fiber~. ~0 g

Greek Chicken

Number of Servings: 4

Time for Preparation: 20 minutes

Time to Cook Recipe: 40 minutes

1 lb~. ~organic chicken breast~. ~boneless and skinless

4~. ~figs

½ c~. ~feta cheese~. ~crumbled

1 tsp. ~. ~salt

1 tsp. ~. ~black pepper

splash~. ~olive oil

Mix the oil, salt and pepper in a bowl. Dip the chicken into it to pick up the flavors of the salt and pepper. Cook in an iron skillet until the chicken is done the whole way through it. When it is done cooking, you will then need to be able to top it with the rest of the ingredients. Serve over a bed of lettuce.

Nutritional Facts:

Calories~. ~369

Net Carbohydrates~. ~7 g

Soluble Fat~. ~18 g

Protein~. ~46 g

Sodium~. ~811 mg

Fiber~. ~3 g

Seared Beef

Number of Servings: 8

Time for Preparation: 10 minutes

Time to Cook Recipe: 60 minutes

4 lb~. ~chuck roast

1~. ~onion~. ~chopped

4~. ~limes~. ~juiced

½ c~. ~cilantro~. ~minced

2 tbsp~. ~garlic~. ~minced

2 tsp~. ~paprika

2 tsp~. ~oregano

2 tsp~. ~cumin

2 tsp~. ~salt

1 tsp. ~. ~black pepper

Use a small amount of organic butter and put it in a large iron skillet. Coat the beef with the rest of the ingredients and put it into the pan. Make sure that it is on medium high heat so that the outside of the beef will get brown. When it is done browning, heat your oven to 400 and cook the meat, in the same skillet, for 40 minutes or until it is tender and juicy.

Nutritional Facts:

Calories~. ~506

Net Carbohydrates~. ~3 g

Soluble Fat~. ~19 g

Protein~. ~75 g

Sodium~. ~733 mg

Fiber~. ~0 g

Pulled Pork No Sandwich

Number of Servings: 8

Time for Preparation: 25 minutes

Time to Cook Recipe: 8 hours

5 lb~. ~pork shoulder

2 tbsp~. ~mustard

2 c~. ~tomato puree

6~. ~dates~. ~pitted and peeled

½ tsp~. ~cloves

½ tsp~. ~cinnamon

2 tsp~. ~salt

splash~. ~olive oil

Put all of the ingredients into a slow cooker. Make sure that they are mixed up well and cook on low for 8 hours. When they are done cooking, take the lid off and use two forks to shred the pork. You can also use a hand mixer to make the shredding easier for you to do. Serve over lettuce or on cloud bread.

Nutritional Facts:

Calories~. ~577

Net Carbohydrates~. ~8 g

Soluble Fat~. ~55 g

Protein~. ~29

Sodium~. ~835 mg

Fiber~. ~5 g

Low-carb Italian

Number of Servings: 8

Time for Preparation: 20 minutes

Time to Cook Recipe: 1 hour

1 lb~. ~ground beef

1~. ~cauliflower head

1~. ~red onion~. ~diced

1 tbsp~. ~garlic~. ~minced

2 c~. ~tomato~. ~crushed

1 c~. ~mozzarella~. ~shredded

1~. ~egg

1 tsp. ~. ~oregano

1~. ~bay leaf

1 tsp. ~. ~black pepper

1 tsp. ~. ~salt

splash~. ~olive oil

Cook your ground beef with your onion and garlic so that it picks up those flavors. In a large casserole dish, combine all of the ingredients together and make sure that the flavors are well combined with each other so that you can use it to be able to put more ingredients in. Heat your oven up to 350 and cook the mixture for 1 hour. Serve hot.

Nutritional Facts:

Calories~. ~342

Net Carbohydrates~. ~8.2 g

Soluble Fat~. ~14 g

Protein~. ~45 g

Sodium~. ~681 mg

Fiber~. ~0 g

Spinacon Chicken

Number of Servings: 4

Time for Preparation: 15 minutes

Time to Cook Recipe: 35 minutes

5~. ~slices of bacon that are fully cooked

2~. ~tbsp. organic butter

1 ½~. ~c spinach

1~. ~tsp garlic, minced

¾~. ~c cream cheese, softened

1~. ~lb chicken thighs

¼~. ~c swiss cheese

¼~. ~tsp salt

¼~. ~tsp pepper

Cook the spinach and the garlic in a large skillet so that they are able to be cooked up. Cut the bacon in small pieces and add it to the spinach and garlic. Put the cream cheese into the mixture and stir it up so that they are fully cooked. Put the chicken thighs flat on a counter or plate and open them up. Stuff the chicken thighs with the mixture that you made and use a toothpick to hold them closed. Put your oven on 350 degrees and cook the chicken for 35 minutes.

Calories~. ~390

Net Carbohydrates~. ~1.2 g

Soluble Fat~. ~21 g

Protein~. ~22 g

Sodium~. ~500 mg

Fiber~. ~4 g

Chicken Tenders

Number of Servings: 4

Time for Preparation: 15 minutes

Time to Cook Recipe: 20 minutes

2~. ~cage free organic eggs

½~. ~c pork rinds crushed

½~. ~c grated parmesan

1~. ~tsp garlic powder

1~. ~tsp onion powder

¼~. ~tsp salt

¼~. ~tsp pepper

1~. ~lb organic chicken breast cut into tenders

Set your oven so that it is at 400 degrees. Line the baking sheet with parchment paper. Put eggs, pork rinds and parmesan along with the seasonings into a bowl. Dip the chicken tenders into the bowl so that you will be able to mix it together and allow it to coat the chicken. Lay each piece out on the baking sheet, do not allow the chicken to touch each other. Cook the chicken for 20 minutes or until the internal temperature reaches 165 degrees.

Calories ~228

Net Carbohydrates~. ~1g

Soluble Fat~. ~8 g

Protein~. ~21 g

Sodium~. ~1380 mg

Fiber~. ~2 g

Chicken Wings, Pub Style

Number of Servings: 4

Time for Preparation: 15 minutes

Time to Cook Recipe: 50 minutes

1~. ~tbsp. extra virgin olive oil

1~. ~tsp salt

½~. ~tsp pepper

2~. ~lb chicken wings

¼~. ~c hot sauce

1~. ~tbbsp melted organic butter

¼~. ~tsp pepper

1~. ~c bleu cheese for dipping

Put your wings on the grill and allow them to get slightly crispy on the outside from the heat of the grill. Bring them inside and put them into a large bowl. Toss them with the rest of the ingredients except for the bleu cheese. Heat your oven to 400 degrees. Put the wings onto a baking dish and cook for 20 minutes. Pull out and flip to cook for another 20 minutes or until they are 165 degrees on the inside. Serve with bleu cheese to dip them in.

Calories~. ~228

Net Carbohydrates~. ~1.7 g

Fat ~17 g

Protein~. ~7 g

Sodium ~600 mg

Fiber~. ~0 g

Pork Chops, Stuffed

Number of Servings: 2

Time for preparation: 15 minutes

Time to Cook Recipe: 20 minutes

2~. ~tbsp. extra virgin olive oil

1~. ~tsp garlic that is minced

3~. ~tbsp. onion chopped

1/3~. ~c spinach

1~. ~egg that has been beaten

¼~. ~c muenster cheese, shredded

2~. ~pork chops

½~. ~tsp salt

¼~. ~tsp pepper

Put the extra virgin olive oil and the garlic into a large iron skillet. Heat up over medium heat and allow it to get fragrant. When it is done, add the spinach to it so that it will wilt. Mix the spinach and garlic with everything else except for the pork chops. When it is mixed, cut the pork chops with a organic butterfly cut and stuff them with the mixture. Put them back into the pan and allow them to get brown on both sides of them. When they are browned, put the pan into the oven and cook at 375 degrees for 20 minutes or until the pork chops are done.

Calories~. ~228

Net Carbohydrates~. ~0 g

Soluble Fat~. ~12 g

Protein~. ~20 g

Sodium~. ~200 mg

Fiber~. ~5 g

Flavorful Brisket

Number of Servings: 14

Time for Preparation: 35 minutes

Time to Cook Recipe: 7 hours

2~. ~tbsp. stevia

2~. ~tbsp. paprika

1~. ~tbsp. garlic powder

1~. ~tsp cayenne

1~. ~tsp salt

1~. ~tbsp. onion powder

1~. ~tbsp. pepper

1~. ~tbsp. chiil powder

8~. ~lb beef brisket

2~. ~tbsp. extra virgin olive oil

1 ½~. ~c beef stock

1~. ~c chopped onion

1~. ~tbsp. liquid smoke

Mix all of the seasonings together with the extra virgin olive oil. Rub that onto the brisket and then place it into the largest slow cooker that you have. Put the beef stock along with the onions and the liquid smoke into the slow cooker with the brisket. Put the lid on and cook it on high for 7 hours.

Calories~. ~342

Net Carbohydrates~. ~8.2 g

Soluble Fat~. ~14 g

Protein~. ~45 g

Sodium~. ~681 mg

Fiber~. ~2 g

Cold Weather Stew

Number of Servings: 12

Time for Preparation: 30 minutes

Time to Cook Recipe: 2 hours

3~. ~tbsp. extra virgin olive oil

2~. ~c diced onions

3~. ~tbsp. garlic minced

2~. ~green peppers diced

2~. ~poblanos diced

2~. ~jalapeno peppers diced

3~. ~lb ground beef, cooked

1~. ~c tomato paste

2 ¼~. ~c crushed tomatoes

1 ½~. ~c diced tomatoes

2~. ~c stout beer

1 ½~. ~tbsp. chilli powder

½~. ~tsp paprika

1~. ~tsp salt

1~. ~tsp pepper

1~. ~tsp cumin

Put all of the ingredients that you have into a very large stock pot. Put it on medium high heat and allow it to cook for two hours.

Calories~. ~150

Net Carbohydrates~. ~1.2 g

Soluble Fat~. ~16 g

Protein~. ~8

Sodium~. ~500 mg

Fiber~. ~6 g

Taco Bowls

Number of Servings: 2

Time for Preparation: 20 minutes

Time to Cook Recipe: 1 hour

1~. ~lb ground beef, cooked

1~. ~can black beans, drained

1~. ~can corn, drained

1~. ~jar salsa

1~. ~packet ranch dressing mix

1~. ~c pepperjack cheese

Put all of the ingredients into a large bowl and mix up so that they are well combined together. When you have done that, transfer them to a casserole dish. Cover and cook for 1 hour or until the ingredients have all melted and gotten hot. Serve in bowls or over a bed of lettuce.

Calories~. ~277

Net Carbohydrates~. ~8 g

Soluble Fat~. ~12 g

Protein~. ~25

Sodium~. ~190 mg

Fiber~. ~13 g

Chapter 10:

Snack Recipes

Rice for Snacks

Number of Servings: 4

Time for Preparation: 15 minutes

Time to Cook Recipe: 20 minutes

1 head~. ~cauliflower

1 c~. ~chicken stock

4 tbsp~. ~organic butter

1 tsp. ~. ~salt

Put the cauliflower into a food processor to make rice the way that you did when you were doing simple no-carb rice. Put the "rice" into a medium sized sauce pan and put the heat over medium. Add the organic butter, salt and chicken stock and let it cook until it is very tender. Serve with some fresh parsley on top of it.

Nutritional Facts:

K Calories~. ~130

Net Carbohydrates~. ~3.5 g

Soluble Fat~. ~13 g

Protein~. ~2

Sodium~. ~635 mg

Fiber~. ~1 g

Mustard Greens with Parmesan

Number of Servings: 4

Time for Preparation: 5 minutes

Time to Cook Recipe: 20 minutes

4 c~. ~mustard greens

2 tbsp~. ~garlic~. ~minced

¼ c~. ~parmesan~. ~grated

1/3 c~. ~almonds

1 tsp. ~. ~salt

splash~. ~extra virgin olive oil

Chop up your almonds into small pieces. Cut the mustard greens so that they are small, too. Mix everything together so that it is well combined and so that you will be able to mix it up. Put it into a small baking dish. Heat the oven up to 350 degrees. Cook for 20 minutes or until it is melted and all combined together well.

Nutritional Facts:

K Calories~. ~140

Net Carbohydrates~. ~4.9 g

Soluble Fat~. ~11 g

Protein~. ~8 g

Sodium~. ~728 mg

Fiber~. ~1 g

Sweet and Savory Radishes

Number of Servings: 4

Time for Preparation: 10 minutes

Time to Cook Recipe: 30 minutes

20~. ~radishes~. ~stemmed

½ c~. ~organic butter

1~. ~juiced lemon

¼ tsp~. ~vanilla

splash~. ~extra virgin olive oil

Melt your organic butter in a sauce pan over medium heat so that it will be able to be used but not to the point where it is completely melted or boiling. Add the radishes and the rest of the ingredients into your sauce pan and then cover them up. Cook for 20 minutes covered, take the lid off and allow it to cook for 10 minutes uncovered.

Nutritional Facts (5 radishes):

K Calories~. ~259

Net Carbohydrates~. ~1 g

Soluble Fat~. ~29 g

Protein~. ~0 g

Sodium~. ~9 mg (unsalted organic butter)

Fiber~. ~0 g

Spicy "Noodles"

Number of Servings: 4

Time for Preparation: 15 minutes

Time to Cook Recipe: 2 hours

1~. ~spaghetti squash

1 tsp. ~. ~red pepper

1 tsp. ~. ~salt

1~. ~lemon~. ~juiced

splash~. ~extra virgin olive oil

Make your spaghetti squash into noodles by cooking it for 90 minutes in a 350-degree oven and then take it out, scrape the insides with a fork so that they go into a bowl and resemble noodles. Mix the noodles up with the rest of the ingredients and put them into a medium sized pot over low or medium heat just so that they can get the flavors mixed together. Serve hot.

Nutritional Facts:

K Calories~. ~75

Net Carbohydrates~. ~5.5 g

Soluble Fat~. ~4 g

Protein~. ~1 g

Sodium~. ~324 mg

Fiber~. ~0 g

BLTC Salad

Number of Servings: 4

Time for Preparation: 20 minutes

Time to Cook Recipe: 60 minutes

1 lb~. ~organic chicken breast~. ~boneless and skinless

2 c~. ~chicken broth

8 slices~. ~bacon

2 c~. ~romaine lettuce

1~. ~tomato~. ~diced

1 tsp. ~. ~salt

1 tsp. ~. ~black pepper

¼ c~. ~mayonnaise

splash~. ~extra virgin olive oil

Flatten your organic chicken breasts using a meat mallet so that they are completely flat. Put the bacon in with the chicken and put the chicken into a small oven-safe dish. Fill about halfway with chicken broth. Cook for 60 minutes or until the chicken is done on 400 degrees. When it is done, take it out and then allow it to sit for a few minutes so that it will cool off. Spread the mayonnaise on top of the chicken and then add tomato with lettuce. Sprinkle the salt and pepper on top of the chicken mixture.

Nutritional Facts:

K Calories~. ~366

Net Carbohydrates~. ~6 g

Soluble Fat~. ~19 g

Protein~. ~43

Sodium~. ~1183 mg

Fiber~. ~0 g

Zucchini Noodles with Sausage

Number of Servings: 6

Time for Preparation: 15 minutes

Time to Cook Recipe: 40 minutes

6~. ~Italian pork sausages

1~. ~onion~. ~diced

2 c~. ~chicken stock

1~. ~tomato~. ~diced

4~. ~zucchini~. ~peeled

1 tsp. ~. ~oregano

1 tsp. ~. ~salt

1 tsp. ~. ~black pepper

splash~. ~extra virgin olive oil

Cook the sausage in with the onion so that it takes in the same flavors that the onion has. When you have fully cooked the sausage, make sure that you chop the zucchini up. Add it all to a small casserole dish and mix it up with the rest of the ingredients so that it is combined together. The flavors will blend better if you are able to mix it up completely. Put your oven on 350 degrees and then cook for 40 minutes on that temperature. When it is done, take it out and serve it hot.

Nutritional Facts:

K Calories~. ~254

Net Carbohydrates~. ~8.5 g

Soluble Fat~. ~14 g

Protein~. ~24 g

Sodium~. ~1049 mg

Fiber~. ~3 g

Warm Salad

Number of Servings: 4

Time for Preparation: 10 minutes

Time to Cook Recipe: 30 minutes

3 c~. ~cabbage~. ~shredded

½ c~. ~walnuts~. ~chopped

¼ c~. ~flaxseed

1 tsp. ~. ~salt

2 tsp~. ~black pepper

splash~. ~extra virgin olive oil

Cook your cabbage in the extra virgin olive oil in a large iron skillet. Make sure that it gets wilty and that you will be able to mix it up nicely. Allow it to cook for a few minutes and then add in the rest of the ingredients. Stir it up and put the cabbage mixture into the oven at 350 degrees for 20 minutes. When it is done, take it out of the oven and immediately top with some extra cheese of your choice or serve how it is.

Nutritional Facts:

K Calories~. ~107

Net Carbohydrates~. ~4 g

Soluble Fat~. ~9 g

Protein~. ~4 g

Sodium~. ~395 mg

Fiber~. ~0 g

The Healthy Dream

Number of Servings: 4

Time for Preparation: 15 minutes

Time to Cook Recipe: o minutes

1 container~. ~sugar free whipped topping

1 block~. ~cream cheese

1 package~. ~gelatin, favorite flavor

1 c~. ~water

Mix the gelatin and the water. The water should be warm but should not be boiling because that will make it harder to use the gelatin. Let the cream cheese soften and then put it in a stand mixer so that it can be fully mixed up. Once it is whipped, fold in the whipped topping. Then, fold the mixture into the gelatin. Top with more of the whipped topping and serve cold.

Nutritional Facts:

K Calories~. ~200

Net Carbohydrates~. ~3 g

Soluble Fat~. ~5 g

Protein~. ~0 g

Sodium~. ~328 mg

Fiber~. ~0 g

Eggs, Devilled

Number of Servings: 4

Time for Preparation: 5 minutes

Time to Cook Recipe: 15 minutes

 5~. ~cage free organic eggs

4~. ~slices bacon, crumbled

½~. ~c mayonnaise

1~. ~tbsp mustard

1~. ~tsp paprika

1/8~. ~tsp salt

1/8~. ~tsp pepper

Cook your eggs in a large pot of water so that they boil for 15 minutes and become hard boiled. Put them into an ice bath and let them sit for 10 minutes while they cool off. Cut the eggs in half lengthwise and then scoop out the yolk so that you will be able to use the yolk. Lay out the eggs. Mix up the bacon, mayonnaise, mustard, salt and pepper in a bowl. Transfer it to a piping bag and then pipe the mixture into the eggs that you have already laid out. When you are done with it, sprinkle just a small amount of paprika on top of the eggs so that they get just a hint of flavor. Serve cold.

K Calories~. ~166

Net Carbohydrates~. ~6 g

Soluble Fat~. ~19 g

Protein~. ~43

Sodium~. ~1183 mg

Fiber~. ~0 g

Chive Rolls

Number of Servings: 2

Time for Preparation: 10 minutes

Time to Cook Recipe: 0 minutes

6~. ~¼ in thick slices of ham

3~. ~oz cream cheese that is soft

1~. ~tbsp chives that are chopped

¼~. ~c Monterey jack shredded cheese

½~. ~tsp garlic powder

½~. ~tsp onion powder

1/8~. ~tsp salt

1/8~. ~tsp pepper

Mix the cream cheese with the chives, the garlic powder, the onion powder, the salt and the pepper. Make sure that they are well combined and that there are no big clumps of cream cheese. Lay out all of the slices of your ham on a platter. Spread the cream cheese mixture on each of the slices of ham. Sprinkle some of the Monterey cheese on top of the cream cheese and roll the ham up. Secure with a toothpick if you are going to be eating later or keep them rolled tightly with plastic wrap.

K Calories~. ~220

Net Carbohydrates~. ~0 g

Soluble Fat~. ~13 g

Protein~. ~22 g

Sodium~. ~800 mg

Fiber~. ~2 g

Buffalo Sauce Chicken Dip

Number of Servings: 8

Time for Preparation: 10 minutes

Time to Cook Recipe: 120 minutes

1~. ~stick of organic butter

1~. ~tsp garlic

4~. ~boneless and skinless chicken thighs

¼~. ~c sour cream

¼~. ~tsp salt

¼~. ~tsp pepper

¼~. ~tsp cayenne

¼~. ~tsp paprika

1~. ~8 oz pack of soft cream cheese

½~. ~c hot sauce

½~. ~c ranch dressing

1~. ~c mozzarella that is shredded

½~. ~c cheddar that is shredded

Cook the chicken so that it is fully cooked the whole way through – grilling works best. When that is done, shred it using a fork or an electric mixer so that you can mix it in with the rest of the ingredients. Use a small slow cooker and put all of the ingredients into it. Stir it up so that they are all well combined and that you will be able to mix all of the flavors together. Put the slow cooker on the low setting and put the lid onto it. Allow it to cook for 2 hours at the minimum and 4 at the maximum. If you want it to be cooked to doneness in a shorter period of time, simply change the slow cooker to the high setting and use the high setting so that you can cook it quicker.

K Calories~. ~331

Net Carbohydrates~. ~2 g

Soluble Fat~. ~9 g

Protein~. ~13 g

Sodium~. ~1600 mg

Fiber~. ~0 g

Chapter 11:

Dessert Recipes

Blueberry Cheesecake Bites

Number of Servings: 16 (bites)
Time for Preparation: 60 minutes
Time to Cook Recipe: 0 minutes

4 tbsp~. ~organic butter

½ c~. ~cream cheese~. ~softened

4 tbsp~. ~coconut oil

4 tbsp~. ~whipping cream

¼ c~. ~blueberries~. ~chopped

1 tsp. ~. ~vanilla extract

Mix up the organic butter with the cream cheese and the coconut oil. The organic butter should be mostly melted before you put it into the mixture. Then, when you are done, you can put the chopped up blueberries into the mixture and then the vanilla. You will then need to whip the whipping cream and then fold it into the rest of the ingredients so that you can create the cheesecake texture that you will be able to enjoy. Put the "cheesecakes" into small reusable cupcake liners.

K Calories~. ~250

Net Carbohydrates~. ~6 g

Soluble Fat~. ~11 g

Protein~. ~2 g

Sodium~. ~428 mg

Fiber~. ~6 g

No Guilt Truffles

Number of Servings: 12
Time for Preparation: 25 minutes
Time to Cook Recipe: 0 minutes

1 block~. ~cream cheese softened

½ c~. ~stevia

2 tsp~. ~coconut extract

½ c~. ~shredded coconut unsweetened

Mix cream cheese and stevia together so that they are well combined together that will make it sweet. Add in the coconut extract and make sure that it is well-combined so that you can make sure that it is all mixed into the flavor. Fold the coconut in and mix it up. Roll the truffles into balls and then put them on a parchment-lined baking sheet. Put them in the freezer for one hour until they harden up When that is done, you can transfer them to the fridge.

K Calories~. ~208

Net Carbohydrates~. ~5 g

Soluble Fat~. ~7 g

Protein~. ~9 g

Sodium~. ~401 mg

Fiber~. ~4 g

Micro Cake

Number   of   Servings: 1
Time   for   Preparation: 10   minutes
Time to Cook Recipe: 0 minutes

2 tbsp~. ~cocoa powder

2 tbsp~. ~stevia

pinch~. ~salt

1 tbsp~. ~whipping cream

½ tsp~. ~vanilla extract

1 egg~. ~beaten

¼ tsp~. ~baking powder

Be sure to use a mug that is safe to go into the microwave because you will be using that to cook this cake. Mix up all of the dry ingredients first in the mug, then add the wet ingredients one by one to the mug. Stir very well with a spoon. When it is stirred up and has no clumps in it, simply put it in the microwave on high for 2 minutes or until it starts to cook. It will bubble up and then it will go back down. You may want to put a saucer underneath incase it does overflow while you are cooking it. Tip: use as large of a mug as possible so that you can avoid the drip problem.

K Calories~. ~169

Net Carbohydrates~. ~4 g

Soluble Fat~. ~12 g

Protein~. ~13 g

Sodium~. ~430 mg

Fiber~. ~8 g

Whips

Number of Servings: 2

Time for Preparation: 5 mins

Time to Cook Recipe: 0 mins

½~. ~c peanut organic butter

1~. ~container sugar free whipped topping, divided in 2

Allow the whipped topping to soften up by taking it out of the fridge around 30 minutes before you are going to make the recipe. In a stand mixer, put the whipped topping and the peanut organic butter or simply use a fork or spoon to mix them together. When the mixture is fluffy, put it into a piping bag and pipe it onto a parchment covered baking sheet. Put it in the freezer for about 2 hours and serve cold.

K Calories~. ~150

Net Carbohydrates~. ~0 g

Soluble Fat~. ~10 g

Protein~. ~12 g

Sodium~. ~110 mg

Fiber~. ~2 g

Raspberry Fat Bombs

Number of Servings: 4

Time for Preparation: 10 minutes

Time to Cook Recipe: 0 minutes

1~. ~c raspberries

½~. ~c coconut oil

½~. ~tsp stevia

½~. ~c organic butter that is melted

Make sure that your coconut oil is melted before you make these. Put all of the ingredients into a food processor and pulse it until they are completely mixed together. The mixture should be a red or pink color. While they are still in liquid form, put them into a silicone ice cube tray. Put the tray in the freezer for 1 hour or until the organic butter and coconut oil get hard again. You can then transfer them to your fridge. Enjoy as a quick snack when you need extra energy.

K Calories~. ~431

Net Carbohydrates~. ~2 g

Soluble Fat~. ~28 g

Protein~. ~4 g

Sodium~. ~1600 mg

Fiber~. ~5 g

Cheesecake

Number of Servings: 4

Time for Preparation: 20 minutes

Time to Cook Recipe: 0 minutes

2~. ~boxes of cream cheese softened

1~. ~tsp stevia sweetener

1~. ~container of sugar free whipped topping

1~. ~tsp almond extract

After you are sure that the cream cheese is softened as much as possible, put it in a stand mixer and make sure that it is whipped completely so that you will be able make sure that it is not clumped together. Add in the stevia and the almond extract to the cream cheese so that it will be able to take on the flavors of it. When it is done, fold in the whipped topping. Divide it into four different ramekins so that you will be able to eat it in different ways. Top with a few raspberries or blueberries and some additional whipped topping for an extra flair or simply serve it plain.

K Calories~. ~381

Net Carbohydrates~. ~0 g

Soluble Fat~. ~7 g

Protein~. ~4 g

Sodium~. ~208 mg

Fiber~. ~5 g

Chapter 12:

Drink Recipes

Green Strawberry Smoothie

Number of Servings: 2

Time for Preparation: 10 minutes

Time to Cook Recipe: 0 minutes

1 c~. ~ice that has already been crushed

½ c~. ~almond milk

2 c~. ~spinach~. ~washed and dried

½ c~. ~strawberries~. ~destemmed

1 tbsp~. ~coconut oil

Put your ice into a blender or a food processor. Pulse it until it is not as chunky as when you first got it when it was crushed. Then, add the almond milk. Make sure that the coconut oil is in the liquid state instead of the solid state. Add the rest of the ingredients to the smoothie in the blender or the food processor. Pulse for a few minutes until there are no chunks of anything. It should be smooth with a few speckles from the very small strawberry seeds. Best if served right away and served cold so that the flavors taste as good as possible and the almond milk does not get sour.

K Calories~. ~201

Net Carbohydrates~. ~5 g

Soluble Fat~. ~8 g

Protein~. ~3 g

Sodium~. ~104 mg

Fiber~. ~6 g

Peanut Organic butter Shake

Number of Servings: 2
Time for Preparation: 10 minutes
Time to Cook Recipe: 0 minutes
1 c~. ~ice~. ~crushed

¼ c~. ~PB2 (or any other powdered peanut organic butter)

¼ c~. ~whipping cream

2 tbsp~. ~coconut oil

1 c~. ~almond milk

Add the ice to your blender first and pour the almond milk on top of it. Push the pulse button on your blender or your food processor so that it will be able to combine the ingredients that you have already put into it. When you have done that, add the rest of the ingredients, making sure that the PB2 is the last ingredient that you are going to put into the mixture. After this, you will need to make sure that you are pulsing it as much as possible and that you are going to be able to use what you can from it. If you want to add an extra layer of flavor, put some unsweetened cocoa powder in it or some dark chocolate nibs.

K Calories~. ~189

Net Carbohydrates~. ~0 g

Soluble Fat~. ~9 g

Protein~. ~14 g

Sodium~. ~801 mg

Fiber~. ~11 g

Coffee Smoothie

Number of Servings: 1

Time for Preparation: 5 minutes

Time to Cook Recipe: 0 minutes

1~. ~c coffee, black

¼~. ~tsp stevia

1~. ~c crushed ice

1~. ~c almond milk

Put all of the ingredients into your blender and pulse it so that they get mixed up together. You may want to allow the coffee to cool in the fridge before you make this recipe so that it does not melt the ice and cause the smoothie to lose the texture that it has in it.

K Calories~. ~239

Net Carbohydrates~. ~4 g

Soluble Fat~. ~5 g

Protein~. ~2 g

Sodium~. ~490 mg

Fiber~. ~0 g

Conclusion

Thank for making it through to the end of *Ketogenic Diet Recipes: 155+ low-carb recipes for weight loss beginners.* Let's hope it was informative and able to provide you with all of the tools you need to achieve your goals of

The next step is to use the meal plans and shopping list to help you prepare for the ketogenic diet and what you will be able to do with the diet.

Finally, if you found this book useful in any way, a review on Amazon is always appreciated!